D1276570

Preschool Stuttering

What Parents Can Do

Series Titles

How to Teach a Child to Say the "S" Sound in 15 Easy Lessons

How to Teach a Child to Say the "R" Sound in 15 Easy Lessons

How to Teach a Child to Say the "L" Sound in 15 Easy Lessons

Preschool Stuttering

What Parents Can Do

Mirla G. Raz

Gersten Weitz Publishers

Published by GerstenWeitz Publishers, 8356 E. San Rafael Dr.,
Scottsdale, AZ 85258

Copyright © 2014 by Mirla G. Raz

Library of Congress Catalog Number: 2013948943

ISBN: 9780963542625

This book is dedicated
to children who struggle to speak fluently
and their parents who struggle to help them.

Contents

Charts

Chapter One

Understanding Stuttering

Starting Points

✓ Psychological problems do not cause stuttering.

✓ Emotional problems do not cause stuttering.

✓ There is no known medical reason for stuttering.

✓ There is nothing a parent has done to cause the child to stutter.

✓ Stuttering, if not addressed, has emotional, social and psychological consequences.

✓ Early intervention is the best prevention.

Introduction

Is it normal for a preschooler's speech to sound choppy? Is it normal for a preschooler to repeat sounds and words? Have you thought that your very normal preschool child sounds like he is stuttering at times? Do all children go through a period of repeating sounds and words? Does my child stammer or stutter? Can stuttering be cured? When a preschooler repeats sounds or words is he stuttering or just doing something normal for his age? Will he stutter for the rest of his life? Is repeating sounds and words a normal part of speech development that the child will outgrow? Is feeling helpless normal for parents? What can parents do to help their child and shed the feeling of helplessness? No matter what parents feel, believe or have been told, ultimately they and their child will benefit from reading this book.

In A Nutshell

There is no known medical reason for stuttered speech in early childhood. Stuttering, or disfluent speech, is not a disease or an illness, nor is it caused by a disease or illness. There are no medicines that will cure stuttering. Psychological and emotional problems do not cause stuttering. There is nothing that a parent has done to cause the child to stutter.

Most children begin stuttering between the ages of two and five years old. Importantly, the preschool years are the prime years for ensuring that a child will not be burdened by a stutter. There will never be a better time. Young children accept change easily. Their self-image has not been affected by their speech, their stuttering has not become a part of them, and the factors that make it worse are relatively easy to change. The older a child gets the harder it becomes for him to gain control of his speech and it takes longer to achieve control. The earlier it is corrected the less impact early stuttering will have on a child's life. As a child gets older, the negative effects of stuttering have a more lasting impact and the prospects of achieving complete fluency decrease so that by the time a child is a teenager, stuttering becomes a chronic disorder. Adults, who stutter, find that they are continually struggling with their speech while trying to cope with the negative effects of stuttering (Cooper).

Parents cannot always fix everything by themselves. There are times when parents need guidance and help. This book was written to guide and help parents navigate the often scary realm of stuttering. One of the goals of this book is to empower parents to help their child. The good news is that by exerting a degree of control over events and factors that can contribute to stuttering, parents can make it easier for the child to control his speech. By now, I have used the word "control" often. One may wonder how one can help a young child to control his speech. Without doing lessons, there are a number of important ways parents *can* help their child. Reading this book is a starting point. By reading this book, parents will better understand stuttering in the preschool years, the emotional aspects of stuttering, the different ways children stutter, how the child's environment and events can affect his speech, what parents can do, and more.

Since stuttering is more prevalent in boys than in girls, the pronouns he, his, and him are used generically throughout the book. However, what is written applies to girls as well.

As you read this book, keep in mind that we all are disfluent at one time or another, some of us more than others. It is important for parents to keep their child's disfluencies in perspective and make sure that the expectations of their child's speech are realistic.

Is the Child Stuttering, Stammering or Is It Just Normal Preschool Speech?

I once met a mother who was having a difficult time dealing with her preschooler's sudden onset of fluency problems. As we talked, I asked her to describe her child's speech. She told me that her son stammers. She emphatically stated that he did not stutter. He stammered. I asked her what a child who stammers does. She said a child who stammers repeats some sounds or words. I then asked her what a child who stutters does. She stopped, thought, and then said, "Well, I guess he repeats sounds or words. But I don't think of my child as a stutterer." It is natural for a parent to not want to think their child is a stutterer. For this parent, the term stammer was preferred. Yet, the two terms are synonymous. "Stammer" is the British term for "stutter."

Normal disfluent speech can be heard frequently in preschoolers' speech. On occasion, a child will repeat a sound or a word. It might happen once or twice a day. The word or sound will be repeated once or twice before the child finishes what he is saying without repeating again. A child, when he is trying to get a parent's attention, may repeat, "Daddy, daddy, daddy."

This is normal and not stuttering. However, "Da da da daddy" resembles stuttering, especially if it occurs a few times a day.

Demystifying Stuttering

Normal speech has fluency to it. We all occasionally stop, repeat a word, or stop in the middle of a sentence and continue on again. But as a rule, those of us who do not stutter have no trouble speaking in a smooth fashion. Stuttering is the interruption of the rhythm, or flow of speech, if it occurs on a frequent basis. There may be periods when a child's speech will be fluent; however, the stutter reappears, sometimes worse than before.

There is nothing mysterious about stuttering. Stuttering is not something that happens to a child nor is he destined to grow up to stutter. It is something the child does. Therefore, the child needs to discover how to control his speech. As stated earlier, many children between the ages of two and five repeat and hesitate. They may stop in the middle of what they are saying, repeat a word, start again, and then finish what they started. The preschool child's speech does not always flow. It can sound choppy. Words and sounds are repeated. This is normal speech for a preschooler, even though it may resemble stuttering. According to the Stuttering Foundation of America, 25 percent of all children between the ages of two and five years of age will stutter at some point. Children under age three and a half are at greatest risk for beginning stuttering. Stuttering, for most children, will peak during the first three months of onset and then decline (Yairi "Epidemiologic"). The percent of children, who will cease stuttering on their own, is about 80 percent. At least 65 percent of preschool children will regain fluency within the first two years of onset (Yairi and Ambrose). Stuttering will remain a long term problem for about one percent of children. More females than males will regain fluency. The Stuttering Foundation's risk factor chart on page 5 can help parents decide if their child is at risk for stuttering. How can we tell which children will stop stuttering and who will not? The answer is: we

Risk Factor Chart		
Place a check next to each that is true for the child		
Risk Factor	**More likely in beginning stuttering**	**True for Child**
Family history of stuttering	A parent, sibling, or other family member who still stutters	
Age at onset	After age 3½	
Time since onset	Stuttering 6–12 months or longer	
Gender	Male	
Other speech-language concerns	Speech sound errors, trouble being understood, difficulty following directions	

do not know. Research to answer this question remains ongoing. Moreover, because it is not known which children will continue to stutter, it is vital that parents know what to do to help their child.

What Causes Stuttering?

As was stated in the introduction, stuttering is not a disease or an illness, nor is it caused by a disease or illness. There is no known medical reason for stuttered speech in early childhood. There are no cures or medicines for it. Stuttering cannot be "caught." Neither emotional nor psychological problems cause stuttering. A child will not begin to stutter because he plays with a child who stutters or he is with an adult who stutters. Stuttering is not learned or acquired through imitation, nor will it "miraculously" disappear. The way in which a mother talks to her child does not cause stuttering (Miles and Ratner). There is a tendency for stuttering to run in families. Two thirds of adults who stutter reported that someone else in their family stuttered. Yet, for most, there is no family history of stuttering. Other than the family link, there is no agreed upon cause of stuttering. Some experts believe that preschoolers stutter because they think faster than they can speak. In trying to speak as quickly as they think, they trip over their words and stutter. There are studies that show that young children are more apt to stutter on longer and more complex sentences (Zackheim and Conture). Another study has found a link between stuttering, temperament and a child's ability to control his emotional reaction to events. The temperament of children who stutter is such that they tend to have stronger reactions to and less self-control in emotional situations (Conture).

Facts about Stuttering

- ✓ According to the Stuttering Foundation, there are over three million adults, one percent of the population, who stutter in the United States and 45 million worldwide.

- ✓ Most adults who stutter are male. Males who stutter outnumber females who stutter four to one.

- ✓ Disfluent children are as bright as fluent children.

- ✓ Preschoolers, who are disfluent, are no different physically, emotionally or psychologically than fluent children.

- ✓ Early intervention is the best prevention.

- ✓ Stuttering is easiest to correct in the preschool years. It becomes harder to correct as the child gets older.

- ✓ If nothing is done to help a child who stutters, and the stuttering continues, there are many negative social, psychological and emotional consequences in store for the child through the school years on into adulthood.

- ✓ People who stutter are self-conscious about their speech. Their self-image can suffer. It can become a handicap which can determine which vocation a person will or will not choose.

✓ People who stutter usually stutter more when talking on the telephone.

✓ People may stutter more when they feel a strong emotion such as when they are nervous, anxious, frustrated, speaking with an authority figure or under stress.

✓ People, who stutter, stutter less when singing or reciting.

✓ Well-known people who have stuttered: Emily Blunt, Byron Pitts, John Stossel, Kenyon Martin, Nicholas Brendon, Hugh Grant, Joe Biden, Winston Churchill, Carly Simon, Bruce Willis, James Earl Jones, John Updike, Marilyn Monroe, Isaac Newton and Ann Glenn (wife of Senator and former astronaut John Glenn) are just a few.

✓ Anxiety and stress do not cause stuttering.

Chapter Recap

✓ **Stuttering is not caused by emotional or psychological problems.**

✓ **Stuttering tends to run in families.**

✓ **Most children start stuttering during the preschool years.**

✓ **Stuttering is something a child does, not who he is.**

✓ **Children who stutter are as bright as other children.**

Chapter Two

Viewpoints and Reactions

Starting Points

✓ Children who stutter do not have more emotional problems than other children.

✓ Learn how stuttering affects a child's self-image.

✓ Children who stutter may act out negatively or withdraw.

✓ Learn the different ways children may stutter.

✓ A child's stutter can vary in severity.

✓ Learn about the secondary characteristics of stuttering.

✓ The onset of stuttering can be gradual or sudden.

How Others View Children Who Stutter

Some interesting studies have described how teachers, school administrators and pediatricians view children who stutter. All of these professionals negatively stereotyped children who stuttered. Forty-four percent of pediatricians felt that children who stuttered were emotionally unstable (Yairi and Carrico). Teachers and school administrators perceived children who stutter as being shy, nervous, quiet, withdrawn and insecure (Lass). Our society stereotypes people who stutter as being more nervous, anxious, fearful, tense, guarded, passive, and insecure than those who do not stutter (Kalinowski, et.al.). Whether one agrees or disagrees with these views, one cannot deny the significant negative ramifications these misperceptions will have for the child as he grows into adulthood. An adult who stuttered sued the National Weather Service after repeatedly being denied promotions despite outstanding work evaluations. The weather service regional director said she did not promote the defendant because of his inability to make rapid-fire judgments, think quickly, and demonstrate leadership ability. Was her decision not to promote a result of negative perceptions of a person who stutters? The person who stuttered certainly felt that way.

It may not be that children who stutter are emotionally unstable, nervous, shy, withdrawn or quiet. But many children who stutter will, as time goes on, become self-conscious about their speech and, therefore, may appear emotionally unstable, withdrawn, shy, nervous or quiet to others.

How Children Who Stutter View Themselves

Childhood is the time when one's sense of self begins to develop. It is the time when we learn to either feel good or bad about ourselves. There are many factors that affect the way in which we view ourselves.

Parents and siblings play a significant role in the development of the child's sense of self. How a child is viewed by his parents will determine, to an extent, how the child views himself. Friends and teachers also have an impact on the child's sense of self. A child will be influenced by the way other people treat him. The way in which a child perceives himself in relation to other children his age will also affect his sense of self. As they get older, children who do not communicate as effectively as other children their age may see themselves as inadequate in this way. Speech is so important in our lives that anything less than normal speech can have negative effects on the child. A study was done on stuttering and nonstuttering children who ranged in age from seven to fourteen. The researchers found that,

> "...stuttering children, even as early as age seven, showed significantly more negative attitudes towards their own communicative abilities than did their nonstuttering peers. This finding may well be the

result of the negative speech experiences that many of the young stutterers went through as a result of their fluency problem. It would seem that their presumed communicative experiences as stutterers have led them to regard themselves as less than competent verbal communicators." (De Nil)

The impact that stuttering has in children is demonstrated in a disturbing study, now called the Monster Study. In 1939, Wendell Johnson, a professor, researcher, expert in stuttering, and someone who stuttered, performed an experiment with a group of children from a Davenport, Iowa orphanage. Twenty-two orphans (among this group were ten children who stuttered) were placed in one of two groups. Half of the children, those placed in the positive therapy group, were praised for their fluency and how well they spoke. The children placed in the negative therapy group were told they were beginning to stutter and were belittled for each speech imperfection. As the study progressed, the children placed in the negative therapy group began to demonstrate negative psychological, social and academic effects soon after the study began. Sadly enough, some children in the negative group continued to have lifelong speech problems.

Different Ways Children React to Their Disfluent Speech

Disfluent speech is one of the many communication problems some young children experience. Preschool children who are unable to communicate effectively can become frustrated. Young children who are frustrated may hit, bite or kick other children. They may throw temper tantrums more frequently than other children. Some children may withdraw, refuse to speak, prefer to play alone or look to the parent to speak for them. Children who have difficulty communicating may appear to be bullies, shy or just plain difficult. In reality, their behavior

can be a reaction to their communication problems. I have seen
children undergo complete personality changes once they are
able to communicate effectively. Once their children no longer
have speech problems, parents have made comments such as,
"He is like a different child," "It is like he took on a completely
different personality," and "He is a much happier child."
The child knows he can now use his communication skills
effectively. Children begin to relate to him differently, more
positively. He begins to feel better about himself.

What Children Do When They Stutter

Before we look at stuttered speech, it might be helpful to look at
normal disfluencies during the preschool years. As was mentioned
earlier, many preschool children are disfluent sometimes. They
may use fillers such as "um" or "uh" or "er" especially when they
are nervous or put on the spot. They say something, hesitate and
then continue on. Repetitions and hesitations occur infrequently,
perhaps once or twice a day. There is no struggle to speak
associated with normally disfluent speech.

Stuttering during the preschool years can occur gradually or
suddenly. Perhaps you had noticed it occasionally but now it
seems worse. Perhaps you had never noticed it before. Perhaps it
seems to come and go. Your child may have been fluent for two
weeks and you felt great relief. But then the stuttering returned.
No matter what the circumstance, it can be very upsetting to
hear one's young child have difficulty saying a word or sentence.
But what exactly is he doing when he stutters? Let us objectively
look at what he does.

There are different forms of stuttering. Generally, speech
pathologists categorize stuttering as repetitions, hesitations,
prolongations or blocks. Some children exhibit what are called
nonspeech behaviors, or secondary stuttering characteristics or
behaviors. Speech pathologists also describe stuttering as being
mild, moderate or severe. The description of the severity of the
stutter is based on how frequently it occurs, the duration of each

episode, if there are secondary behaviors associated with it, and the degree to which the stuttering affects the child emotionally, academically, and/or socially. Let's look at different types of stuttering in more detail.

Repetitions

- ✓ Repetitions are the most common of all stuttering patterns.

- ✓ Repetition of a sound usually occurs on the first sound of a word. For example, a child might repeat the "g" in the word "go" so that he says, "Gggggggggggo."

- ✓ Repetition of a syllable usually occurs on the first syllable of a word. For instance, a child would repeat "mo" in the "mommy" so it sounds like this: "Momomomomommy."

- ✓ Repetition of one syllable words is common. An example of a word repetition would be, "My my my my my toy."

- ✓ Repetition of multiple words can occur such as "I want I want I want I want to go."

- ✓ Frequent interjection and repetition of "um," uh," "like," "well," and other such fillers as in the following sentence: "The dog um um um is uh uh barking."

A child may repeat a unit one or more times. As a rule, any one or combination of the above, if done frequently, will cause a child to sound like he is stuttering. Any of the above may also occur with a rise in pitch.

Prolongations

A prolongation is the stretching of a word or sound beyond its normal length. For instance, holding the "s" sound in the word "see," so it comes out "sssssee" is a prolongation. They may also occur with a rise in pitch.

Blocks/Hesitations

A block/hesitation occurs before a word is said. A child may tell you that the word gets stuck in his throat or that the word will not come out. Perhaps when he says the word he seems to push it out. It may be that the child's lips quiver or there is noticeable tension in the area of the mouth or throat.

Secondary Stuttering Behaviors

Secondary stuttering behaviors are body or facial movements that a child does before or during stuttering. These behaviors may show up after a child has been disfluent for a few months. In his struggle to speak, a child may blink his eyes, tap his feet, move his eyeballs sideways, raise his upper lip, tilt his head, jerk his head or have visible lip, facial or jaw tension. These are just a few examples of nonspeech behaviors. There are others. You may notice a different behavior as he struggles with his speech. I once worked with a little girl who jerked her head so severely that it caused her to fall off her chair.

Mild Stutter

A mild stutter is characterized by a pattern of occasional sound, syllable or word repetitions. Mildly stuttered speech occurs a few times during the day. There is no struggle associated with speaking. The child does not appear bothered by it.

Moderate Stutter

A moderate stutter is characterized by repetitions of sounds, syllables, words, and/or word groups. A person with a moderate stutter may also prolong sounds or block. Moderately disfluent speech occurs many times during the day. The child may show signs of unease or frustration. He may seem as if he is struggling with his speech.

Severe Stutter

A severe stutter is characterized by the frequent repetition of sounds, syllables, words, and/or word groups. Prolongations and blocks may be evident as well. Severe stuttering occurs every few sentences or on nearly every sentence. You may notice secondary stuttering characteristics. Speaking has become an effort as the child struggles to speak. The child may tense up when speaking, change words, or stop speaking altogether.

Chapter Recap

✓ Stuttering can affect a child's behavior and self-image.

✓ Repetitions are the most common type of stuttering during the preschool years. However, a child may also prolong sounds or words or block/hesitate.

✓ Secondary characteristics can occur and are varied.

✓ There is a range of severity to stuttering.

Chapter Three

Stuttering and Emotions

Starting Points

✓ Children react differently to their stuttering than their parents do.

✓ Parents should not feel responsible for their child's stutter.

✓ Observing the child is important.

✓ Know the wrong ways that adults try to help the child.

✓ Learn what to say and what to do to help the child.

✓ Understand the importance of listening to the child.

✓ How parents talk to the child can make a difference.

✓ Understand how emotions can make stuttering worse.

The Emotions of Parents

I can think of no other childhood speech or language disorder that arouses stronger emotional reactions in parents than stuttering does. What is it about stuttering that hits such an emotional nerve? One answer is that, as parents, we understand the negative social, emotional, psychological, and occupational consequences in store for an adult who stutters. Obviously parents do not want their children to be burdened all their lives by a stutter. Aside from projecting into the future, what is the relationship between the parent's feelings and her preschooler's feelings when he stutters? An article in the American Journal of Speech-Language Pathology helps us understand why parents feel the way they do when their children stutter. The authors write,

"Parents have difficulty clearly differentiating between their feelings about the stuttering and the children's experiences. For example, the parent may be anxious about children speaking to others, but may project this by talking about the child's anxiety in speech situations. In these situations, the parents are feeling emotional distress and projecting the distress onto the children's situation" (Zebrowski). In other words, parents who feel anxious about their children's disfluencies believe that it is the child who feels anxiety when he stutters. The reality is that most very young children do not feel anxious when they stutter. The authors also highlight the different perceptions that parent and child may have about the child's stutter. They state, "In many cases the parents presume that their perspective of the problem is the children's perspective. For example, when children start to notice their own speech disfluencies, they may primarily note this as a difference between their speech and the speech of other children. The parents, on the other hand, may take the perspective that the children's disfluency represents a loss or a disorder. In this way, the parents are defining the experience with a negative connotation that can stimulate intense emotional responses (e.g., anxiety, depression, anger); in contrast, the children may have a more neutral cognition about the situation." In other words, your child may not yet be bothered by his disfluencies. You, however, may feel terrible about them.

Considering the strong parental reactions to stuttering, parents may feel that they have done something to cause their child to stutter. Studies show otherwise. Results of studies of parent-child interactions have shown that,

> "No one behavior has been observed to be uniquely exhibited by parents of children who stutter as opposed to parents of children who do not. In the same vein, no single parental behavior or environmental characteristic has been determined to be 'necessary or sufficient' for stuttering to develop in children. It appears that stuttering in children emerges as the result of a complex

interrelationship between children's inherent and learned abilities and characteristics (speech, language, psychosocial, temperament) and the ways in which the environment (parents) and children themselves respond to these abilities. Stuttering is neither purely constitutional nor purely environmental, and this realization on the part of the parents can be an extremely powerful aid in their attempts to manage feelings of guilt about children's stuttering." (Zebrowski)

If you have been feeling responsible for your child's disfluencies, the results of the above study should help put those concerns to rest. Starting now, it is important to move the focus away from the past and the feelings you may have about the problem to positive ways of helping your child.

Taking the Time to Understand the Child Who Stutters

In order to better understand what your young child is experiencing during this phase, try, for a few minutes, to imagine yourself as a three-year-old. Ready? Let's start:

You are feeling quite good about yourself. You can do a lot of things that you see your mom, dad, and big kids doing. Walking is a breeze and you can run pretty fast. You can throw and kick a ball. You know how to hold a crayon and color in a coloring book. You might even know a few letters of the alphabet. You know how to yell and scream. You also know that if you lay on the floor, kick and scream, you will get someone to pay attention to you. However, by age three, you are probably learning that lying on the floor, kicking and screaming may also get you into big trouble. You know how to talk pretty well. You can even say most of your sounds just like a big person. You know the names of the most important toys and your best friends. When you want something, you use sentences. Actually your sentences are getting longer with each passing month. Yes, you are talking just fine. Then suddenly one day you have trouble saying an easy word. You were just starting to say something and you said, "I" three times in a row. Well, maybe it is nothing. Then it happens again. But this time you had trouble saying more words when you were telling your mom about your car. The next thing you know you have trouble getting your words out smoothly a lot of times. You do not hear big people talking like this. Your mom says her words smoothly. What is happening?

As a parent, you notice the change in your child's speech. What you do now is critical. As your child tries to figure out how to regain control of his fluency, your reaction can make his job easier or can hamper his efforts. At this point, it is important to make some careful observations. Are there situations where his speech is better or worse? Does he speak better with certain people and worse with others? Does his speech get worse when he is anxious, excited, afraid, frustrated or stressed? Observe him, his environment and other people around him when he is disfluent. Jot your observations down on the Information Record on Page 85. We will be discussing places, people, and emotions that can affect your child's fluency in future chapters. What you observe now will be useful later.

Helping the Child Who Stutters

It is natural for parents to want to directly help their child when they hear him stutter. They do so with the best of intentions. In their attempts to help their child, they may give him advice or ask him to do what they believe will help. However, the advice they give can be counterproductive. Advice can make the child more self-conscious and upset with himself for being disfluent. Advice can frustrate the child when the advice does not help and yet the parent believes it will. Numerous adults who stutter have told me that they believe the advice their parents gave them, when they were children, did more harm than good. The advice made them more self-conscious and inhibited.

The list, on the following pages, highlights common advice that should be avoided, why the advice should be avoided, and replacement actions the parents can implement that will be more beneficial. It is also shown as Chart One on p. 89.

Do's and Don'ts

Avoid Saying or Doing: "Say it again," "Say it again this way," or "Say it the way I say it."

Reason: You do not want the child to feel that how he talks is wrong or that he is bad because he is disfluent. Also, saying it again does not insure that the next time will be better.

Instead Say or Do: Listen to what your child is saying. Respond to what he said, not how he said it.

Avoid Saying or Doing: "Speak slower," "Slow down," or "You are talking too fast."

Reason: The child's speaking rate is not going to determine whether or not he will stutter. (Rapid speech and strong emotional reactions are issues that should be dealt with on their own and not in relation to stuttering, at this point. If the help of a speech pathologist is sought, she will consider these issues as she plans a therapy program.)

Instead Say or Do: Listen to what your child is saying. Respond to what he said, not how he said it. Focusing on rate of speech will not eliminate a stutter. The child, if he knows what you mean by slowing down, will simply speak slower and stutter. The child will need to learn to control his speech. As he struggles with his speech, he may discover that slower speech allows him greater control over how he speaks. As he learns control, he may slow his rate on his own.

Avoid Saying or Doing: "Think before you speak" or "Think about how you are talking."

Reason: Thinking before speaking will not eliminate a stutter. Should the child think about what he wants to say or how it should come out?

Instead Say or Do: Listen to what your child is saying. Respond to what he said, not how he said it.

Avoid Saying or Doing: "I am not going to listen to you if you talk that way."

Reason: It is extremely important that the child feels that what he has to say is important. It is important for a child's self-concept and his desire to improve his communication skills. Refusing to listen to a child because he stutters can convey the idea that what he has to say is not important unless his speech meets a fluency standard. What a child has to say is important no matter how it is said.

Instead Say or Do: Listen to what your child is saying. Respond to what he said, not how he said it.

Avoid Saying or Doing: "Every time you talk that way you will get punished."

Reason: If a child is disfluent, he has not figured out how to control this aspect of his speech. If he cannot yet control his disfluent speech, but he can control whether or not he speaks, your child may avoid speaking in order to avoid a punishment. Speech avoidance is not uncommon among children for whom stuttering has been a problem. You do not want your child to avoid speaking since that can lead to other issues.

Instead Say or Do: Listen to what your child is saying. Respond to what he said, not how he said it.

Avoid Saying or Doing: "Calm down." "Relax before you talk."

Reason: Children do not stutter because they are not calm or relaxed. True, stuttering can increase when a child feels a strong emotion. But strong emotions contribute to, rather than cause, the problem. Important are the reasons for the strong emotions. Advising the child to calm down or relax before talking focuses attention on the stuttering without discovering the cause of the strong emotions. There have been children who have told me that such advice made them so angry, they stuttered more as a result.

Instead Say or Do: Listen to what your child is saying. Respond to what he said, not how he said it.

Avoid Saying or Doing: "Take a deep breath before you talk."

Reason: By saying this you are suggesting to the young child that deep breathing before talking helps him to avoid stuttering. Untrue. A deep breath before talking may distract the child the first couple of times resulting in a fluent start. However you may find that the child takes a deep breath and stutters anyhow. There is also the risk that the instruction may lead to a block. The child may take a deep breath, hold it and then push out the word. Or, it may become a secondary stuttering characteristic. In other words, the child may begin to believe that he cannot talk fluently without taking a deep breath. As a result, he may take a deep breath before he says anything, becoming an attention grabbing behavior on its own.

Instead Say or Do: Listen to what your child is saying. Respond to what he said, not how he said it. Avoid giving him advice.

I worked with a preschool boy who stuttered moderately. He was making nice progress in therapy. One weekend his parents went out of town and his grandparents came into town to take care of him and his sister. When he came to our first therapy session, after that weekend, he could barely speak. He continually gulped for air as he tried to speak. It was a wonder he did not hyperventilate. During our session, I was able to learn from him what had happened. To "help" him stop stuttering, his grandparents had instructed him to "breathe" before he talked.

Avoid Saying or Doing: "Stop talking that way."

Reason: Since children and adults do not stutter on purpose, it is not helpful to tell them to stop.

Instead Say or Do: Listen to what your child is saying. Respond to what he said, not how he said it.

Avoid Saying or Doing: Speaking for your child or finishing words or sentences no matter how strong the urge.

Reason: This can be very frustrating for the child.

Instead Say or Do: Listen to what your child is saying until he is done. Then respond to what he has said.

Avoid Saying or Doing: Interrupting your child when he is speaking.

Reason: Interrupting the child is disruptive and can be frustrating. It was found that parents of children who stutter interrupt their children more often than do parents of children who do not stutter (Kasprisin-Burrelli, et al).

Instead Say or Do: Listen to what your child is saying until he is done. Then respond to what he has said.

When a child who stutters is interrupted or interrupts another person, he usually stutters more than if there is no interruption. A study was done to determine how conversational turn-taking affected the speech of a five-year-old boy who stuttered. The results of the study showed that when conversational turn-taking was instituted, the five-year-old's stuttering decreased. When the turn-taking rule was ignored the child stuttered more (Winslow).

Avoid Saying or Doing: Speaking for your child to help him or because you are embarrassed by his speech or you believe he is.

Reason: Children can sense when their parents feel bad or are embarrassed by what they are doing. Your child may feel worse about his speech if he senses your discomfort.

Instead Say or Do: Allow your child to speak and complete his thoughts on his own. Do not help him or speak for him.

Avoid Saying or Doing: Facial or body language shows that you are anxious or upset when your child is talking.

Reason: Sometimes facial expressions can convey as much information as words.

Instead Say or Do: Listen calmly and patiently to your child. Make sure that your facial expression does not convey a negative emotion about how he is talking.

Avoid Saying or Doing: Asking your child to perform or recite in front of other people.

Reason: There are children who dislike performing on the spot.

Instead Say or Do: Proudly tell others what your child can do without asking him to perform or recite.

Avoid Saying or Doing: Talking about your child's speech to other people while he is present.

Reason: The child may be embarrassed that you are talking about him. The exception is if you are talking with the speech pathologist who will work with your child.

Instead Say or Do: Speak to the other person at a time when the child is not present.

Avoid Saying or Doing: Getting upset or distressed when your child is disfluent.

Reason: Seeing a parent distressed or upset because he has stuttered can make a child feel bad.

Instead Say or Do: Listen unemotionally to how your child has spoken. Express your emotions to what he has said rather than how he has said it.

Avoid Saying or Doing: Calling your child a "stutterer."

Reason: Stuttering is something the child does, not who he is. This period in your child's life does not define him.

Instead Say or Do: Accept your child as he is without labeling him.

Avoid Saying or Doing: Limiting the amount of time your child has to speak.

Reason: Time pressure can result in an increase in stuttering.

Instead Say or Do: Allow your child to say what he would like to say no matter how long it takes.

Avoid Saying or Doing: Bombarding your child with questions.

Reason: It can be overwhelming for anyone to respond to many questions at once.

Instead Say or Do: Calmly ask your child a question and patiently wait for the answer. Keep questions short and simple. Respond to what your child has said before you ask another question.

Avoid Saying or Doing: Poking fun of your child's speech by imitating or teasing him.

Reason: This behavior can result in a range of emotions. The child may avoid talking.

Instead Say or Do: Listen to what your child has said without commenting on how he has spoken.

How Emotions Affect the Child's Fluency

Adults who stutter are able to describe the emotions they feel, and from them we have come to better understand the relationship between emotions and stuttering. Adults, who stutter, say that their stuttering gets worse when they are nervous, scared, anxious, angry, frustrated, excited, intimidated, stressed out or when speaking with an authority figure. Even those of us who do not stutter know that our speech can be affected when we feel a strong emotion. Children are like adults in this way. If a child feels angry, nervous, afraid or frustrated, he may become disfluent. It is important that parents be aware of the emotions that can result in an increase in stuttering. Understanding the impact of emotions will enable parents to help the child through the disfluent phase in his speech development. Below is a short list of the emotions that often result in an increase in disfluent speech.

Frustration

There are numerous reasons a young child may feel frustrated. I have highlighted instances when a child may feel frustrated and how the parent can help the child:

- ✓ A child may get frustrated when they are trying to do something that is too hard for him. Try to make the task easier if you see your child getting upset. A child will readily accept change in a task that allows him to succeed.

- ✓ A child may get frustrated if he feels that nothing he does is good enough to please. Make sure you accept the child's limitations and are reasonable in your expectations. Try to avoid criticism. Instead of focusing on what he cannot do, focus on what he does well. Praise the child for the things he tries to do as well as for the things he succeeds in doing.

- ✓ A child may get frustrated if a parent does not listen to him. When the child talks, give him your undivided attention. Do not interrupt him or finish his words or sentences for him. When he is finished talking, respond to him in a way that makes him feel that what he said has significance.

- ✓ A child may get frustrated if he has difficulty communicating. Children who are difficult to understand

and children whose stutter is moderate or severe can experience frustration. Unfortunately, for the disfluent child, stuttering and frustration become a vicious circle. The child wants to say something, has difficulty getting his words out and becomes frustrated, which results in greater difficulty getting the words out fluently. Listen patiently as the child struggles and avoid giving advice. Respond to what he has said and not how he has said it. When the child has said something that is difficult to understand, one can rephrase what one thinks the child has said. For instance, if the child said, "Uh uh uh uh wan pay wegos," the parent can say, "You want to play Legos?" If that is not what the child meant, it may be necessary to ask the child to show the parent what he wants. Once you know what it is, it is important to verbally acknowledge his statement by saying, "Oh, you want _____." Remember to also respond to what the child has said.

Anxiety

Children may feel anxious when they anticipate that something out of their control will happen. Below, I have outlined times when a child might feel anxious:

✓ A child may feel anxious if he does not like where he is going. If a parent notices that the child does not like going to a particular place, the parent should try to find out why. If your child states a specific reason for not wanting to go, address the reason. For example, perhaps the child does not want to go to daycare or preschool because another child hits him. Parents should do what they can to remedy the problem.

✓ A child may feel anxious if he does not want to be with someone. If a parent notices that the child does not like someone or does not want to spend time with a person, the parent should try to find out why. If the parent is able to determine the reason, she can try to find a solution for the child. If the reason cannot be determined, it may be best not force the child to spend time with the person.

✓ A child may feel anxious if his usual routine is disturbed. A change in routine can include vacations, change of school, teacher, caretaker, the absence of a family member or a move to a different home. Parents can talk about the upcoming change with the child. The child's concerns should be addressed, if possible in a positive light.

✓ A child may feel anxious if he feels he may have done something wrong. He might get that message if one's voice is raised or one sounds irritated. Facial expressions, a raised eyebrow or worried look may send a message that can make a child anxious. Parents should try to talk calmly with the child, if he has done something wrong.

Excitement

It is common for young children to repeat and hesitate when they feel excited. They are so enthusiastic and eager to tell about why they are excited that they may lose control of their speech. Parents can help the child by doing the following:

1. Stop what you are doing.

2. Lower yourself to eye level with your child.

3. Assure your child that you are listening.

4. Without mentioning his speech, tell your child that you can see he is very excited.

5. Ask your child to tell you what happened. Listen, without interrupting, until he has finished. Do not comment on how fluent or disfluent he was.

6. Do comment on what your child has just told you.

Stress

Children may feel stressed when they are pressured to do more than they are capable of at the time or there are many demands made of them. Below are times when a child may feel stressed and some suggestions for helping the child:

- ✓ A child may feel stressed if he knows a task is too hard for him. Know the child and his capabilities. When asking the child to do something, be sure that he is capable of succeeding at the task.

- ✓ A child may feel stressed if he feels he never does anything good enough. Let the child know what a good job he is doing and how pleased you are with him. Once again, focus on what he can do rather than on what he cannot do.

- ✓ A child may feel stressed if he is involved in too many activities. Soccer, swimming lessons, learning a musical instrument, gymnastics, ballet, karate, and cooking classes are wonderful activities. However, too many activities can be overwhelming and stressful for a child. Along with the input of the child, select one or two activities for him to participate in during the week. Leave the other activities for another time.

- ✓ A child may feel that he is being pressured to perform or live up to his parents expectations. Parents are naturally proud of their children and their accomplishments. We see our children as reflections of ourselves; if they do well, maybe we feel that we look better. Sometimes this translates into a form of competition, with our children as the competitors. The upshot is one may expect one's child to be able to do certain things for which he may not be ready. For instance, a parent may want to teach her three-year-old the alphabet. The child may not be interested because he is not ready. If the parent persists, the child can feel pressured. The end result is likely to be an increase in stuttering. Parents can try to break down tasks into separate steps so that success comes easier for the child. As an example, if the child needs to clean up his toys, the

parent can ask him to put his Legos in the box. Once the
Legos are in the box, he can be asked to put his trucks in
the basket. These two steps would take the place of asking
the child to clean up his toys.

Fears

Children have fears of all kinds of things we long ago learned
were silly. However, to a child these fears are real. When the
child appears afraid or says he is afraid, listen to him. The child
looks to the adult for comfort. Discuss his fears with him. Think
of ways to help him deal with them. Think of how to make what
he is afraid of look harmless. For instance, let us say the child is
afraid or dogs. Below are suggestions for helping the child:

✓ *Read children's books about the fear*: Read children's
   illustrated books about dogs.

✓ *Try to change the child's negative thoughts by using positive
   words*: When talking about dogs use positive descriptions
   like dogs are fun, they help people who cannot see, the
   bark to help people know someone is at the door, they like
   to play, they can protect people and they can be someone's
   best friend.

✓ *Confronting the fear in steps*: Introduce the child to a puppy.
   Before doing so, tell the child that the puppy may get
   excited and jump on him but that is okay. If the child is
   hesitant to approach the puppy, try a gradual introduction.
   Slowly try to close the distance between the child and
   the puppy. This can be done during the visit or over a few
   days.

✓ *Talk and Role Play*: Tell the child that it is important to
   let a dog smell his hand before he touches the dog. One
   might say, "Dogs have really good noses. They know who
   people are when they sniff them. Hold out your hand like
   this (demonstrate) before you touch a dog. After he sniffs
   your hand you can pet him softly." Then role play the

above using a stuffed animal. Perhaps the parent wants to make-believe she is the puppy.

How Parents Can Help Their Child
The Importance of Listening

When we talk to someone, we like to feel that that person is paying attention to us. A listener conveys attentiveness through eye contact, body language, and verbal responses. In our culture, good listeners make eye contact with the speaker. Eye contact and body language tell the speaker that he/she has the listener's attention. A verbal response lets the speaker know that he has been listened to. When a child recognizes that an adult is not listening, he may repeat the same thing over and over again. Also, knowing that the listener is not tuned in can be frustrating. Frustration, as has been discussed, is one of the emotions that contribute to fluency problems.

I cannot stress enough the importance of being a good listener. Adults expect children to be good listeners. When we talk to them, we expect them to listen. They are taught to be good listeners in school because good listening skills are vital for academic success. Yet, in the rush of a normal day, many parents do not listen when their children are talking to them. It is not that we do not want to listen. It is simply that children may talk when the parent is busy doing something. When they talk, parents may half-listen. Half-listening is continuing to do what one is doing, not making eye contact with the child, and responding in short one-word answers, hoping that the answer will be satisfactory. Or, instead of half-listening we do not listen at all. The child knows we are not listening because he has said "Mommy," "Daddy," or what he has on his mind a few times in an attempt to get our attention. The result, for the child can be frustration, anxiety, feelings of stress or perhaps believing that he is not important, any of which can lead to an increase in stuttering.

Below are suggestions for improving one's listening skills:

✓ Stop what you are doing.

✓ Lower yourself to the child's level.

✓ Make eye contact with the child.

✓ Wait until the child has finished speaking. Do not interrupt him no matter how disfluent his speech may be.

✓ Ignore stuttered speech.

✓ Do not finish the child's sentences for him.

✓ Respond to what the child has said not how he has said it.

✓ Do not walk away from the child as he is talking.

✓ If other children are present, signal them to remain quiet until the child is finished talking to you.

✓ Ignore mobile devices.

Mobile devices have become ever-present in our lives. We rely on them for a host of reasons. Their benefits are numerous but there are downsides to our reliance on these devices. One of the major downsides, that I have observed time and again, is the way that they draw attention away from children with whom the adult should be engaging. I have lost count of the number of times I have witnessed adults ignoring children while they talk, text or play with their smartphones or tablets. When parents are with their child, I would suggest turning off or ignoring the phone or tablet.

Talking With Your Child

Parents are the child's most important people. It is important that the child feels comfortable talking to his parents.

Now is the time to lay the groundwork for a comfortable talking relationship.

Before we get into the "hows" of talking with the child, parents can ask themselves this important question, "Do I enjoy talking with my child?" I hope the answer is yes. If, however, the answer is no, it is important to figure out why. Is it because you do not feel you have the time? Is it because you do not have the patience? Is it because your parents never talked to you and you feel you turned out okay? Whatever the reason, now is the time to turn over a new leaf. Work on learning to enjoy talking with your child. Notice that I wrote "Talking *with* your child," rather than, "Talking *to* your child." When you talk with the child, you will be conversing rather than telling him to do something or scolding him if he has done something wrong. When talking with the child, it is important to show interest in him and what he has to say. Parents can show interest by stopping what they are doing to listen and, when the child is done, responding to him. It is important to look at the child. One may want to hold his hand or put one's arm around him. One's voice should be calm and indicate patience. One's volume should be normal. Speaking loudly, may give the child the impression that the parent is angry. One's rate of speech should be normal. Speaking quickly may make one hard to understand. Rapid speech may make the child feel that the parent is in a hurry and does not have the time to talk. Rapid speech may make the child feel pressured which, in turn, may result in an increase in stuttering (Guitar et al).

Parents should try shortening and simplifying their sentences (Guitar et al). For example, a sentence such as, "You need to take a nap now because otherwise you will be tired when John comes over to play with you later this afternoon," is lengthy and complex. The child may be overwhelmed by the amount of words coming at him. One can easily simplify the sentence by breaking it down into two sentences such as, "You are tired. You need to take a nap before John comes." Simplifying one's speech may take some practice but one's efforts can help the child.

The words one chooses and facial expressions are also important. Parents should be aware that if one looks concerned, worried or anxious those emotions will be conveyed to the child.

In summary when talking with your young child:

✓ Speak in normal volume and at a normal rate.

✓ Take your time when you talk.

✓ Keep your sentences short and simple.

✓ Your attitude should convey the message that you want to talk with your child.

✓ Select positive words when talking with your child.

✓ Get down to your child's level physically.

✓ Smile, relax, and be patient.

Special Time

Special time allows the child to have positive and uninterrupted time with his parent. Special time should be relaxing. The individual attention the child gets from his parent can have an indirect positive affect on stuttering.

Parents should try to spend ten to twenty minutes interacting with the child. Special time should not be used for correcting the child's speech. This time should not be interrupted by electronic devices or other family members. Phone calls can go unanswered or the caller can be told he will be called back. If that is not possible, one can give the child something to do and tell him dad will be right back. Try to keep the phone conversation short. Special time should not be interrupted by other children either. The time should be devoted to giving attention only to one child. Other children can be told that they will get their special time in a little while.

In two parent households, whoever is at home during the day, should try to give the child special time during the day.

The parent who is not home during the day should set aside special time before the child goes to bed. If neither parent is home during the day, parents can alternate evenings for special time. It is important to arrange the day or evening so that the parent is able to give the child his/her undivided attention. Both parents need to make the effort because the child has different, yet important, relationships with each parent.

There are many things a parent and child can do during special time. Mobile devices and computers are particularly appealing to children. Children enjoy playing board games with an adult. Reading books is fun. Children have wonderful imaginations. Parents can play school, alien invasion, restaurant, doctor or whatever the child chooses.

Chapter Recap

✓ **Parent should take care not to convey negative emotions about the child's stuttering.**

✓ **Neither parents nor their parenting skills have caused the child to stutter.**

✓ **Unhelpful advice can be replaced by positive actions.**

✓ **The emotions that can make stuttering worse are: frustration, anxiety, excitement, stress, and fears.**

✓ **The way in which parents listen and talk to the child can make a difference.**

✓ **Care should be taken not to allow the cellphone, and other forms of modern technology, to grab parental attention away from the child.**

Chapter Four

Different Environments, Events, and People

Starting Points

✓ Learn about how Ordinary Magic can enhance the parent/ child relationship.

✓ Learn how the home environment can impact the child.

✓ Learn the ways to make it easier for the child to be fluent at home.

✓ Understand how the child's preschool and/or daycare can impact the child's speech.

✓ Learn how to assess whether the child's preschool is appropriate for him.

✓ Know what events can affect a child's fluency.

✓ The cooperation of siblings is important.

✓ Learn what to ask of teachers and caregivers.

✓ Know what to say to relatives, other adults and children.

The Home

When I work with a preschooler with fluency problems I get to know the parents and how they relate to their child. I try to understand the child's relationship with family members and his home environment.

The quality of child-parent relationships—interactions and attachments—has been found to be extremely important in the dynamics of stuttering. A recent study examined different patterns of parenting between families of children who stutter and those who do not stutter. It was found that caring, warm, less demanding and less authoritarian parenting styles contributed to fluency. Demanding, authoritarian parents and lack of parental warmth impeded fluency (Beilby). This is not to say that a lack of rules and discipline is good. Rather, it is important that children have rules to follow and that parents be consistent in their discipline without being authoritarian. The rules should apply to all the children in the household. At the same time, parents should be warm and caring towards all their children and favoritism should be avoided. Ultimately, the parents should strive for what is called Ordinary Magic. The term applies to parenting in general. The goals are:

- ✓ For the child to manage impulsivity
- ✓ Fewer positive rewards (children should perform tasks not for a tangible reward such as a toy)
- ✓ Structure within the home
- ✓ Positive attachment
- ✓ Discipline
- ✓ High Autonomy (allowing a child to gain confidence by doing for himself)
- ✓ Self-regulation (example: learning to control emotions such as anger)
- ✓ Self-management of behavior (example: learning not to tantrum)

Keeping Ordinary Magic in mind, I describe four different types of home environments. The descriptions are general and may not completely apply to any one home. However, parents may be able to find similarities between their child's environment and those discussed. None of the environments cause a child to stutter. However, certain environments can negatively impact a child who does. See if any elements in the homes described apply to yours. If your home contains elements in the homes described, consider what was recently discussed and try to make the changes suggested. I think you will find that even small changes will make a difference in your child's fluency.

Home A–The Chaotic Environment

✓ There is a lot going on at once.

✓ The television is playing even though no one is watching.

✓ There is loud music playing even though no one is listening.

✓ Family members need to yell to be listened to or heard.

✓ The adults feel pressured to get things done and are rushed when interacting with the child.

✓ The adults speak rapidly.

✓ One or both parents feel stressed and have little patience left for the children.

✓ There is little discipline and the parent(s) may feel out of control.

✓ Children feel they must fight with their siblings for their parents' attention.

Home B–The Perfectionistic/Strict Environment

✓ One or both parents are perfectionists and expect the children to be perfect at all times.

✓ The house is immaculate and must be kept that way.

✓ The child must always look neat, clean, and well-dressed.

✓ The parent(s) is/are rigid in what the children may or may not do. There is little tolerance for children who do not meet the parents' expectations as to proper or improper behavior.

✓ The parents may post a list of "bad" behaviors and punish the child for any deviation.

✓ The parents offer little warmth and comfort to their children.

✓ The children may feel uncomfortable discussing their feelings or problems with the parents.

Home C–The Hostile Environment

✓ The children in this home can never do anything right. They are viewed as lazy, stupid, and/or mean.

✓ The children are frequently punished for even minor mistakes.

✓ The parents argue a lot with each other and the children.

✓ The children are blamed for problems the parents may have.

✓ The children are given many responsibilities and have little time for themselves.

✓ The children are made to feel incompetent no matter what they do.

✓ Cursing and yelling occur frequently.

✓ Household members rarely smile at the children or voice approval of them.

✓ The parents offer little warmth or comfort to the children.

✓ Parents resent being interrupted in their activities.

Home D–The Balanced/Calm Environment

✓ The television plays only when someone is sitting and watching a particular program.

✓ When music plays it is at a volume that does not compete with anyone who may need to talk.

✓ Family members are involved in one activity at a time.

✓ Family members do not compete for space when involved in an activity.

✓ Family members speak in normal speaking voices and use a normal speaking rate.

✓ Family members do not need to compete with one another to be heard. Each person feels that he will be able to talk when it is his turn.

✓ The parents do not place demands on the child that are excessive.

✓ The parents understand that young children get messy and dirty, and make messes. Children are not punished for being children.

✓ The parents praise their children.

✓ The parents enjoy their children and let their children know they are loved.

✓ Children are given autonomy appropriate to their age and gain confidence in their abilities.

✓ The home is generally calm and relaxed.

The balanced environment, although not ensuring a child will not stutter, may at least reduce the emotional components that can contribute to stuttering. If your home is more like Homes A, B or C, some tweaking may be helpful. Here are some general suggestions:

✓ Get rid of ambient noise. For instance, if the television is playing and no one is watching, turn it off. The same thing goes for other electronic devices. In other words, turn off unnecessary distractions.

✓ Reduce the amount of activity in the home. Parents may
find themselves doing a few different things at once.
Here is a possible scenario: It is five o'clock and you start
preparing dinner. The toddler wants to cook too, so the
parent gives him some pots and spoons. While the dinner
is cooking and the child is playing, the parent decides to
get some ironing done. While the parent is ironing the
phone rings or a text message comes in. The child notices
the parent is busy with the phone and comes over to tell
her something, but the parent is in the middle of telling/
texting the caller something. The child says, "Mommy"
nonstop until the parent tells the caller to hold on a
minute. The parent may feel somewhat irritated and
asks the child what he wants. He tells her that he needs
something else to cook with. The parent puts the iron
down and tells the caller to hold on a minute. Suddenly
something is boiling over on the stove. The parent forgets
about the child and rushes to the stove. Once the stove
crisis is handled the parent remembers that the caller is
still waiting. The parent returns to the caller. The parent
is no sooner back to the phone and ironing when the child
is nose to nose with the parent again.

   If the above scenario sounds familiar, it would be
helpful to reduce the amount of activity in the home.
If you are cooking, do not add another activity such as
ironing. While the food is cooking, and if you have spare
time, help your child "cook" with the pots and spoons you
gave him. By doing this you are giving your child valuable
attention and quality time. If the phone rings or a text
comes in, tell the caller/texter you will call back. If the
call is important, try to be brief.

✓ Everyone deserves his own space. If too many people are
trying to do their activities in the same space, chaos may
ensue as people start getting in each other's way. Let's
go back to the kitchen scenario. The parent is preparing

dinner and gives the toddler pots and spoons to play with. Chances are, if left to decide where to play, he will plant himself, along with his pots and spoons, right at his parent's feet. Instead of handing him the pots and spoons, the parent can place the pots and spoons in a nearby space and tell the child that this is a good spot for him to cook.

✓ Speak in a normal speaking voice (volume). It is important to assess whether family members speak to each other at a normal volume. For some reason, there are families who have gotten into the habit of yelling at home. They have become so accustomed to using a loud volume that they are not aware of how loud they sound. Such families may also not be aware that because they are loud they may sound angry. If a child feels that his parents are angry he may feel anxious, fearful or stressed.

✓ Studies have shown that when parents, who tend to speak rapidly, talk slower to a child the child's fluent speech increases (Starkweather, Guitar). Parents who speak rapidly should make a conscious effort to slow down. If a parent speaks too rapidly, she may, without even realizing it, make the child feel as if he is a bother or intruding on his parent's time. The reasons, underlying rapid speech, may also be factors that can affect a child's fluency. Is the parent always rushing to do things? Does he not wish to be interrupted? Do they feel that there is never enough time to get things done? Does she feel pressured at work and/or at home? Additionally, people who speak too quickly can be harder to understand.

✓ Sometimes there can be talking time rivalry among siblings. Parents should work on allowing each person his own talking space. In other words, if someone is talking, others wait until he is finished before responding. Also, family members should not interrupt the speaker. Ask that each child wait his turn without interrupting the person who is speaking.

✓ Perfectionism places tremendous stress on children. Parents should not expect the child to do things perfectly. It is hard for many of us to live up to a perfectionist's expectations.

✓ Work on making your home relaxed and calm. If the child is experiencing temporary fluency difficulties, a calm, relaxed environment will make it easier for him to regain control of his speech, by reducing the emotional catalysts of stuttering.

✓ Be consistent with discipline but not overly rigid and demanding. The child should know what to expect from his parents and the demands should be within his ability to accomplish. The rules should be clear. A behavior that he was punished for today should not go unpunished tomorrow. Parents should be consistent in disciplining their child and should not disagree in front of him about what to do about his behavior.

✓ Be consistent in routines. There is security for a child in being able to predict what needs to be done and when. If a child is in childcare, arrangements should be made to bring him there and pick him up at the same time. I am not an advocate of once a week or every now and then placement in a childcare facility. A child needs to feel he is a part of a group. It is hard and stressful for a child to make friends and establish himself as part of the group if he attends sporadically.

✓ If the child is still napping, naptime should occur at the same time each day. Putting the child down for a nap at a time that is convenient for the parent may be difficult on the child. If he does not have a routine, he may resist napping unless he is exhausted. If he is exhausted, he may be cranky as well. Exhaustion and crankiness can result in an increase in disfluencies.

✓ Set a reasonable bedtime hour for your child and establish a bedtime routine. Try not to keep the child beyond his bedtime. It is harder for a child to control his fluency if he is tired and a tired child is more likely to stutter. A bedtime routine, such as taking a bath then reading a book together, can help a child get ready for sleep.

✓ Do not show more leniency or strictness to the child who stutters, than one shows to other family members.

✓ Try to eliminate sibling rivalry. Do not compare children or show favoritism. Give each child your undivided attention. The children should not have to compete with each other for your time or approval. One way to reduce competition for attention is to set up special time each day for each child. Talk, play or read with each child for ten to thirty minutes daily.

✓ Let your child know he is loved no matter what he does. Praise, hugs, and kisses go a long way in conveying the message that your child is loved.

Preschool and Daycare

It is important that parents visit their child's preschool at different times of the child's day to observe the environment in which he plays and learns. Parents should observe how the adults interact with the children and how the children interact with each other. Parents should watch their child and see how he interacts with the adults and other children. If he is disfluent, how do the adults and children react to him? There are other factors to consider as well. Below is a list with negative and positive attributes to look for in a child's program. It is also shown as Chart Two on p. 94. Negative attributes observed should be discussed with the classroom teachers as well as what can be done.

What to Look for in the Child's Preschool

Negative Attribute: The environment is noisy.

Positive Attribute: Children and adults use their "indoor" voices. If music is playing, its volume is low.

Negative Attribute: Children are walking or running around aimlessly.

Positive Attribute: Children are engaged in activities and the adults are engaged with them.

Negative Attribute: You observe children pushing, pulling, hitting or kicking other children or teachers.

Positive Attribute: Children are respectful of one another and "use their words" instead of resorting to negative physical contact.

Negative Attribute: Children are sitting around with nothing to do.

Positive Attribute: Children are playing or talking with one another.

Negative Attribute: There are too few adults in the room for the number of children.

Positive Attribute: The ratio varies with the age of the children. There should be fewer children per adult for younger children. Check your state's guidelines.

Negative Attribute: There are a lot of people in the room. Overcrowding is a problem.

Positive Attribute: The room is large enough to accommodate the number of people in it.

Negative Attribute: The caregivers are inattentive to the children and their needs.

Positive Attribute: The caregivers are focused on the children and engaged with them.

Negative Attribute: The caregivers look grumpy or frazzled.

Positive Attribute: The caregivers should look happy.

Negative Attribute: The teachers use criticism when talking to the children.

Positive Attribute: Teachers should use positive words and be generous with praise. When a child has done something wrong, the teacher should ask the child to say what he has done that was wrong. The teacher should ask him how he could have handled the problem differently and assist him as needed.

Negative Attribute: Teachers swap classrooms during the day reducing the children's consistency with caregivers.

Positive Attribute: The children have the same teachers throughout the day, every day.

Negative Attribute: The school has a high teacher turnover rate.

Positive Attribute: The school retains the same teachers throughout the year.

Negative Attribute: Children tease one another.

Positive Attribute: Children are respectful of the other children.

In summary, parents should expect their child's preschool or daycare environment to have a low noise level, be calm, warm, and stable. Additionally, the adults should be nurturing, positive, and attentive to the children and their needs. Parents who feel that their child's preschool environment is not the best can first try speaking to the teacher or primary caregiver. Explain that your child is presently experiencing fluency difficulties. You understand that fluency difficulties are normal for children your child's age and that there may be other children in the room who are experiencing similar difficulties. Parents who feel changes are in order can also set up an appointment to meet with the director of the preschool or daycare center. They can talk with her about what was observed in the child's room and the changes they feel would be beneficial. After speaking to the child's teacher and the school director, parents should wait a few days and return for an unannounced visit. Has the teacher or daycare provider made the recommended adjustments? If yes, great! If nothing has changed, it may be necessary to look for a different daycare center or preschool.

Events That Can Affect Fluency

It is not unusual for children to stutter more when their routine is disrupted or changed. Some events can be fun and exciting while others can be stressful. Some may appear minor while other events can have a meaningful impact on the family. The increase in stuttering can last a few hours, until the event is over, or it can last a few days, if the child's emotional level is still high.

Special Holidays and Events

Holidays and special events are times of excitement. Even the anticipation of a big celebration is exciting. People are busy getting ready, buying gifts, arranging schedules, and traveling. Perhaps we move faster and talk faster getting ready for something special. The turmoil of holidays or special events can affect a young child. Parents may find that their child's disfluencies increase at holiday time or before, during, and following a special event. Parents can anticipate an increase in disfluencies and should try to remain calm. During these periods, parents should monitor their speech and make sure they are not talking too quickly or loudly. Schedules and routines should be kept as normal as possible. During these special times, it is important that parents take the time to listen calmly and patiently to their child.

Fatigue or Illness

Children's disfluencies can increase when they are tired or sick. Pediatricians recommend that preschoolers gets at least 10-12 hours of sleep each night. Children may need more sleep at night if they no longer nap during the day. Parents may also notice an increase in stuttering when their child is sick. This should not be a cause for alarm. Once the child feels better, parents can expect the return to his pre-illness fluency level.

Divorce or Separation

Witnessing friction between parents is an emotionally difficult experience for children. Divorce or separation of parents can cause anxiety, frustration, stress, and fear to come together in one package. The probability is high that a preschooler will become more disfluent prior to, during, and soon after a divorce or separation. Parents can help their child get through this difficult period by getting the child to talk about his feelings and carefully listening to what he says. Parents should make an effort to respond with care and understanding. If the child feels that he did something wrong, assure him that he did nothing wrong. Parents should make it crystal clear to the child that he did nothing to cause the problems between the parents. Reassuring him that he is loved and spending some extra time with him can go a long way in helping him regain fluency. It is also important that the parents agree on how to help their child deal with this difficult event. It is in the child's best interest if both parents talk with him. Parents should be in agreement about what to tell him and how it should be done. A child who receives different messages can become confused as to which parent he owes his loyalty. It is important to recognize that the child is not getting divorced from his other parent. He must be made to feel that his loyalty to each parent will remain the same. Conflicting messages can cause the stress, frustrations, and fears of this difficult time to become magnified and, as a result, the disfluencies may greatly increase in frequency and severity. It also may be advisable to seek the help of a child counselor or psychologist.

Death or Illness

A death or serious illness in the family is a trauma that can cause emotional upheavals in a household. It may be difficult for parents to put up with the trials and tribulations of raising a young child when they are upset. As a result they may find that they have less patience for their child. Or, they simply may not have the time to spend with the child. A young child may not understand what is happening but he will see that the parents are upset or have less patience or time for him. During this trying time, parents may find that the child's stuttering has increased. Parents can help their child by talking with him about why they are sad, upset or busy. They can assure him that soon everyone will feel better. If possible, parents should try to set aside some time each day just for him. If that is not possible, try the following: Get a large calendar. Show the calendar to the child. Select a day within the next three or four days, not longer. Draw a happy face on that day. Show the child the happy face and tell him that, on that day, you and he will spend time together. Then cross out the date that you have started the count. Thereafter, with the child at your side, cross out each day as it passes. For example, if it is Sunday and you plan to spend time with your child on Wednesday, put a happy face on Wednesday and place an X in the Sunday box on the calendar. On Monday place an X in the Monday box. Do the same on Tuesday. Since time concepts are difficult for children to grasp, a calendar will help your child visualize and anticipate your time together.

Financial Problems

Money is another issue that can cause strife in family interactions and routines. Young children will be aware of a problem because they will notice changes in their parents' behavior towards each other and perhaps other family members. As we have discussed throughout the section, changes can result in an increase in disfluencies. At this trying time, it is important that parents assure their child that they are not upset with him. They should try to keep the family routine as normal as possible. When parents interact with their child, they should try to keep their concerns about their financial situation locked away temporarily, as if they were momentarily nonexistent.

New Baby

A new brother or sister means changes for the family. Parents will have less time to spend with their other children. They may not be as patient as they were before the baby arrived. They may be too tired to give their preschooler the time he needs. The net effect of a new baby, on a preschooler, can be an increase in stuttering. Or, out of the blue, he starts stuttering. Once the parents understand the dynamics of stuttering, this change can be expected. The child is going through a period of emotional upheaval as well as being drawn into the excitement of the new addition to the family. Yet, he may feel stressed by the changes needed to accommodate a new baby. He may feel frustrated and angry that he receives less attention or that he has to share his parents with another person. Perhaps he is afraid that, with all the time and attention the baby gets, his parents love him less.

One way to lessen the disturbance of a new baby, is to prepare the child for the arrival of his sibling. Parents should explain to their preschooler what it will be like having a new baby around. They should talk to him about how things will change and how things will remain the same. Parents should reassure him that their love for him will never change, even though they will be busy with a new baby. If the baby has already arrived, parents can talk to their preschooler now about what is happening, why things have changed and what he can expect to happen over the next few weeks.

Once the baby has arrived, parents should try to set aside a half-hour of uninterrupted attention each day for their preschooler. This is his special time with his parent. Parents should make an effort to have special time at the same time each day. This way their preschooler can anticipate his special time and look forward to it.

Other Events

Moving, changing the primary caretaker and changing schools/daycare facilities can affect fluency. When a change is anticipated, parents can help by preparing the child.

There are different ways parents can prepare their child. Visiting the new house, school or daycare facility is a good way to introduce the child to what will be his new surroundings. If possible, view the new site a few times before the move takes place. In this way, the child can get accustomed to how the site looks visually. If visiting the new home or school is unlikely, show the child pictures and talk about them. When workable, try to arrange visits to a new school. The first visit can be short, just for the child to see the school from the inside and his new room. Another visit can be longer with the child and parent staying in the room together. On a subsequent visit, perhaps the child can stay an hour or two, without the parent. If the child will have a new caretaker at school or at home, talk to the child about why _____ is leaving and who the new person will be. Talk about how the person looks or if available show him a picture of the caregiver. Perhaps the new caregiver can visit the home a couple times before starting the job. Some children can be eased into the change by drawing pictures of the new house, school or the new people that will come into his life.

Talking with the child about the changes that will take place can help ease the adjustment. What parents say should put the changes in a positive light. Below are some suggestions.

✓ The new house or apartment will be bigger so the child will have his own room.

✓ The house or apartment will smaller so the child's room will be closer to the parent's room.

✓ A park will be nearby.

✓ The child will get to make new friends.

✓ They will live closer to the child's school.

✓ The school has fun toys.

✓ The teachers are very nice.

✓ The new caretaker is a good cook.

✓ The new caretaker knows a lot of fun games.

Help Others Help the Child
Siblings

The impact that stuttering has on a child's siblings should not be underestimated. Siblings can feel guilt, resentment, loss, negative emotions, and greater closeness towards their brother or sister who stutters. Some have expressed feelings of rivalry for their parents' attention. Yet, siblings have expressed a desire to be involved in helping (Beilby et al). It is important to acknowledge that their brother is talking differently than the way they talk. Parents can start out the conversation by saying, "I know that your brother is taking a long time saying his words. That may be frustrating for you. But I would like to ask you to help out," or "Your brother is learning to say his words smoothly. There are many ways you can help your brother." Parents should ask their nonstuttering children how they feel about their brother's speech. To demystify stuttering, parents should explain that many children, when they are young, repeat words and sounds. Sometimes learning to talk can be like learning to walk. Young children trip and fall a lot until they get good at walking. Sometimes, they repeat words and sounds until they get good at talking.

Below are what older siblings can be asked to do to help their brother:

✓ They should never tease their brother about the way he talks.

✓ They should not mimic their brother's disfluent speech.

✓ They should not tell their brother how to talk.

✓ They should not say things like, "Slow down," or "Watch how I talk."

✓ They should not finish words or sentences for their brother.

✓ They should not talk for their brother.

✓ They should not laugh when their brother is having difficulty saying words.

✓ They should not call their brother names like stupid, retarded or dumb.

✓ They should try not to frustrate or get their brother angry on purpose.

✓ They should not interrupt him when he is talking.

Parents should emphasize the helpful things they can do such as:

✓ They should be good listeners when their sibling talks to them. Explain that being a good listener means they stop what they are doing, look at their brother as he talks to them, and listen quietly. Parents can help their children by giving them a "signal" that it is time to be quiet and listen to their brother.

✓ Wait patiently until their brother has finished talking. Explain to your children that each person must wait until the person who is talking is finished. Tell them that each of them will get a turn, but they must wait quietly until it is their turn.

Teachers and Daycare Givers

It is important to talk to the child's teachers, babysitters, and daycare providers about the child's speech. If they have worked with many preschool children, they should know that disfluent speech is a part of normal speech development. However, they may not know how to deal with a child who stutters. Or, perhaps they feel they have methods that are helpful. Regardless, it is vital that the parents speak with them and tell them how they want the staff to deal with their child's problem. Parents should arrange for a parent-teacher conference where they talk about his speech and the importance of everyone working together. Below are some points to stress with the child's teacher or daycare giver:

✓ It is important that the child feel that the teacher/caretaker is listening to him. The teacher should get down to his level, make eye contact, and give him the opportunity to say what is on his mind.

✓ Ask the child's teacher not to give him advice as to how to talk.

✓ Ask the teacher to allow him to finish what he is saying without interruption.

✓ Ask the teacher to allow him to finish what he saying without help. She should avoid finishing words or sentences for him.

✓ Ask the child's teacher if there is any child with whom the child does not get along. If there is, request that the teacher do what she can to keep the two from interacting until the child passes this disfluent stage.

✓ Share the child's fears with the teacher. Ask the teacher to avoid placing him in a situation that may make him fearful.

✓ Generally, two- to five-year-old children do not tease or make fun of one another. However, if there is a child who teases or makes fun of the child's speech, ask that the teacher speak with that child about stopping the behavior.

I recommend that the child's teacher/caregiver read this book in order to help her better understand preschool stuttering.

Relatives and Adult Friends

Well-meaning relatives and friends may offer parents advice on how to handle the child's disfluencies. If you or any of your brothers or sisters went through a disfluent phase as young children, your parents may tell you how they handled the situation and that it worked. After all, you or siblings are, in all probability, fluent adult speakers. At times, relatives or friends may take it upon themselves to give the child advice as to how he should talk. They may advise him to, "Slow down," or "Think before you talk," or offer other words of advice. Parents can explain, to concerned relatives and friends, that they have learned helpful ways of dealing with their young child's disfluencies. Parents should explain that they can help best by simply listening, without comment, when the child talks to them. They should stop what they are doing, get down to the child's level, make eye contact, and listen. They should not interrupt the child nor should they finish his words or sentences for him. Ask that they accept the child's disfluent speech just as they accept his fluent speech.

Other Children

We know that there are children who tease other children. Parents should speak privately to the child who is doing the teasing. They should calmly explain that some children have trouble getting their words out. One can acknowledge that their child talks differently by saying, "I know that _____ is taking a long time saying his words. That may be frustrating for you. But I would like to ask you to help out," or "_____ is learning to say his words smoothly. There are many ways you can help him." Parents may add, "Maybe there were times when you had trouble getting your words out." Parents can ask the child for his help. They should explain how he can be a good listener when the child speaks to him and how important it is that he listens to what the child is saying and not how he says it.

Below are what other children can be asked do to help:

- ✓ They should not tease _____ about the way he talks.

- ✓ They should not mimic _____'s disfluent speech.

- ✓ They should not tell _____ how to talk.

- ✓ They should not say things like, "Slow down," or "Watch how I talk."

- ✓ They should not finish words or sentences for_____.

- ✓ They should not talk for _____.

- ✓ They should not laugh when _____ is having difficulty saying words.

- ✓ They should not call _____ names like stupid, retarded or dumb.

- ✓ They should try not to frustrate or get _____ angry on purpose.

- ✓ They should not interrupt him when he is talking.

Chapter Recap

✓ Ordinary Magic has been shown to have a positive impact on the parent/child relationship.

✓ Although the child's home environment does not cause stuttering, it can impact the child.

✓ Speaking in a normal volume and not rapidly can help the child.

✓ Making changes in the home environment can help the child regain fluency.

✓ It is important to determine if the child's preschool is the best one for him.

✓ Holidays, special events, financial problems, separation or divorce, fatigue, illness, the death of a loved one, a new baby, moving, or a change of caregiver can impact the child's fluency.

✓ Engaging the cooperation of siblings, teachers, caregivers and other significant adults is important.

Chapter Five

Professional Help

Starting Points

✓ Know when professional help may be necessary.

✓ Learn what qualifications to look for in the search for a speech pathologist.

✓ Know the important questions to ask the speech pathologist.

✓ Know the important information the professional will need from the parent(s).

✓ Learn what it takes for therapy to succeed.

Intervention May Be Needed

I hope this book has given you a better understanding of the dynamics of early childhood stuttering and has removed some of the mystery that often surrounds this speech problem.

Now you will need to take the information and use it to your child's benefit. As you have learned, it often takes more than a wait and see attitude for a child to "outgrow" a problem. Parents need to be proactive if they are to help their child "outgrow" stuttering.

Parents need to beware of physicians, preschool teachers, and speech pathologists who tell you your child will outgrow the problem. Although about 80 percent of disfluent preschoolers will stop repeating sounds, syllables, and words, there are a small number that will continue to stutter into adulthood if not helped. A study was done to determine the percentage of children, age three to eight, who still stuttered after receiving a stuttering diagnosis and recommendation for therapy, but received no therapy. Sixty-two percent of the parents had not enrolled their children in therapy because they had been told by a professional that their child would "outgrow" the problem. It was found that the majority still stuttered six to eight years after the problem was originally diagnosed. Some children's stutter had gotten worse (Ramig).

Today is the day to start doing whatever it takes to help your child. Once you have adopted the suggestions and made the necessary changes discussed in this book, give yourself a few months to see what happens. Hopefully your child will not need professional help. However, there are some children who will need professional intervention from a speech pathologist. The investment you make in professional therapy early on will be worth every dollar.

When to Seek Professional Help

When trying to decide when to seek professional help, parents should keep in mind that a preschooler is still young and time is on his side. I say this because I understand the emotional impact that stuttering can have on parents. Below I have listed guidelines that parents can use to decide when to seek professional help.

✓ The child has begun to exhibit what are called secondary stuttering characteristics. Secondary stuttering characteristics are unusual movements a child makes during disfluent moments. Some common secondary characteristics are eye blinks, facial tics, head jerks, quivering lips, and covering his mouth with his hands.

✓ Parents have followed the guidelines discussed in this book but their child continues to stutter six months later.

✓ The child avoids speaking or speaking situations.

✓ The child has turned five years old and is still stuttering.

✓ Parents disagree on how their child's disfluencies should best be handled even after having read this book.

✓ A parent's level of anxiety is too great for him or her to deal unemotionally with the child's stuttering problem.

✓ One or both parents feel that speaking with a professional will make them feel better.

Where to Get Professional Help

A certified or licensed speech pathologist is the person most qualified to help you and your young child. Most states require a speech pathologist to be licensed. Once you have selected a speech pathologist, you should ask her if she is licensed. You can verify licensure by asking to see her license or by calling your state's Board of Medical Examiners. You will know if a speech pathologist is certified if she has the letters C.C.C. after her degree. These letters stand for Certification of Clinical Competency. Certification is given by the American Speech-Language-Hearing Association (ASHA). A speech pathologist is certified only after she has completed her Master's degree, several hundred hours of clinical training, a clinical fellowship year, and passed a rigorous exam. She must also maintain her membership in ASHA to maintain her certification status. A certified speech pathologist will present her credentials as follows: Mirla G. Raz, M.Ed., CCC-SLP.

I recommend that you seek out a certified or licensed speech pathologist who works primarily with children and has worked successfully with children who stutter. You can find local speech pathologists, in private practice, by asking your child's teacher or pediatrician to recommend someone. (The Physician's Checklist, put out by the Stuttering Foundation, on page 98 can be copied and given to the child's pediatrician and teacher for them to complete.) ASHA and the Stuttering Foundation have the names of speech pathologists, in your state, who work with individuals who stutter. The ASHA website for finding

a professional near you is http://www.asha.org/findpro. The
Stuttering Foundation website is http://www.stutteringhelp.org/
referrals-information.

Comparing Speech Services in the Public Schools and Private Practice

A child who stutters may be eligible to receive speech therapy
for free from the local school district. A federal law, the
Individuals with Disabilities Education Act Amendments
of 1997 (IDEA, P.L. 105-17) mandates that state education
agencies and local school districts provide special education
services to children ages 3-21 who need them in order to receive
a free, appropriate public education (FAPE). Speech therapy
is considered to be special education. Even though IDEA
is designed to provide a free, appropriate public education,
children attending private schools are covered under the
law too. There are several differences in how the services are
provided but even if your child attends a private school, he may
be eligible to receive free speech therapy from the local school
district. Preschool children, who stutter, are eligible for these
services if they are shown to have an educational disability. It
is important that you understand that a speech problem does
not necessarily qualify a child to receive speech services. Be
prepared to demonstrate that your child's speech is handicapping
him. The speech problem must be shown to have a significant
negative impact on the child's education so that it can be
considered to be an educational disability. This will need to be
determined by the school speech pathologist. She may
want to know how well he socializes and expresses his needs and
feelings. Some questions she may ask are: Does the child avoid
speaking with other children or adults? Do other children avoid
playing with him? Does he refuse to speak at home or in his
preschool class?

Getting therapy for a child in the public schools is a process.
First, the parent must contact the public schools and tell them

about their child's problem. The district will want the child to be screened by a speech pathologist in the district. Once the child is screened, a decision will be made whether the child's problem is severe enough to warrant testing or if the child should be rescreened next year. If the decision is made to test, the child must be tested within a specified amount of time following the screening. If the testing finds that the child is not eligible for services, the parent will be asked to monitor the child's progress until next year. If the child's speech problem meets the criteria for eligibility for services, the professional will write the child's goals for the year in an Individualized Education Plan (IEP). This entire process can take three months or more.

Public school services run on a school calendar year. When school is not in session, your child will not have speech therapy. This interrupts progress. Your child may be fortunate to have a half-hour of individual therapy. As a rule though, therapy is provided to small groups of two to five children of different ages with different speech problems. The sessions are a half-hour for all children in the group. You can determine how many minutes of therapy your child gets by dividing 30 minutes by the number of children in the room. Thus, two children would get 15 minutes of therapy each, three children 10 minutes and so on. Perhaps your child's therapist schedules two half-hour sessions for your child each week. All too common is the once weekly therapy session. The public school's speech pathologist is the one your child will work with; parents have no choice in the matter.

If you decide to seek therapy with a speech pathologist in private practice, you can select someone who is experienced working with preschool children who stutter. The evaluation should take no more than an hour. The decision to start therapy can be made then or on the subsequent visit. You will see the professional each time you bring your child in for therapy and you can ask about the child's progress during the session. With private therapy, your child will be seen individually for the entire session. Therapy will be more consistent because private therapy does not run according to the school calendar. Therapy is year round and can be scheduled for two or three sessions a week. This allows for greater consistency in therapy and faster progress.

Regardless of where the child will receive therapy, once you have committed to therapy, it is important to make it a priority. It should be more important than sports, dancing lessons, music lessons, etc. There are good speech pathologists in the public schools and in private practice. I know how appealing free can be. But consider that free services can cost more in the long run if the problem is not treated in a timely fashion. This is your child's future and that should be the priority.

> The experience of one parent:
>
> In my child's case his speech delay was not "severe" enough to be accepted into the speech program at the public school. A year later, a sudden onset caused him to not be able to get words out at all. We had to seek immediate therapy. I wish I had followed my instincts and sought outside therapy when he was younger. I think it's important for parents to understand that the public school system is inundated and sometimes, even when your child does require therapy they may tell you it's okay when your child really could benefit from therapy.

Paying for Therapy and Health Insurance

Some states have programs that cover for speech services for children with disabilities from birth to 36 months of age. Parents can contact the state agency that provides services for children with developmental disabilities.

Private therapy can be costly. However, I suggest that one think of it as an investment in the child's future the cost of which will only go up as the child gets older. This is because waiting beyond the preschool years means therapy will take longer. As children get habituated to their speech pattern, the longer it will take for therapy to change it. Thus, it is important to make therapy a priority financially and time-wise. Speech pathologists understand that the cost of therapy can be a difficult for some parents. The speech pathologist may have a sliding scale. If she does, she may want to see the parents' tax returns to determine how much to discount therapy. Some speech pathologists offer a payment plan. The parent can discuss what the family can afford to pay for each session. The parent and speech pathologist can then agree to a schedule of weekly or monthly payments to be paid, once therapy has concluded, until the remaining balance is paid off.

It is worthwhile to review one's policy or contact a health insurance representative to ask about their coverage for speech services. Ask the health insurance representative if they cover for *evaluation of speech fluency* and therapy for *childhood onset fluency disorder*. They may want codes for these services. The CPT code for *evaluation of speech fluency* is 92521 and the diagnostic code for *childhood onset fluency disorder* is 315.35. If one's health insurance does provide coverage, it is important for the parent to ask the representative to specify the limits of coverage. Some health plans cover for the evaluation and therapy, others for only the evaluation, others for only therapy, there may be monetary caps and so on. It is important to get the name of the health plan representative with whom you talked and ask for confirmation of coverage in writing as well as any limit on the number of sessions, co-payments, deductible amounts, etc. The health plan should provide this written notification within 30 to 60 days. Some insurance companies require that there be a medical reason for the speech problem. In that case, it may help to provide the health plan with information about the neurological basis of stuttering. Parents can point out that children who stutter have demonstrated atypical brain anatomy and that deficits in this network for speech production may represent risk factors for the onset of childhood stuttering. (Chang et al).

Another avenue for parents, who need financial assistance, is to contact a local civic organization such as the Elks Club, Lions, or Rotary.

What to Expect When Seeking Professional Help

What the Speech Pathologist Will Want to Know

- ✓ She will want to know about the child's speech and language development and general health.

- ✓ She will want to know when the problem was first noticed and by whom.

- ✓ She will want to know how constant the problem has been.

- ✓ The speech pathologist will ask each parent his/her perceptions of the problem.

- ✓ She will want to know when the child's speech is better and worse. Each parent will have something valuable to contribute so that the speech pathologist can gain more insight into the child's problem by understanding his home environment and family dynamics.

- ✓ She will probably want to know how each parent relates to the child and how each deals with his disfluencies.

- ✓ She will want to know how the parents relate to each other and how well they get along.

✓ If the child has brothers or sisters, she will want to know their ages, how they get along, and how they are disciplined.

✓ The speech pathologist will want to know if the child goes to preschool and when. She may, at a later date, wish to visit the preschool and meet the teacher.

The cooperation of the parents and the information they provide is vital to the success of the therapy program. Therefore, it is best for the parents to be forthright in their responses.

A speech pathologist working to help a disfluent preschooler will work closely with the family. Based on what she learns from the interview she will be able to tailor therapy to achieve fluent speech more rapidly. At some point, she will involve the parents in the therapeutic process. She will suggest ways for the parents to help their child.

Important Questions to Ask the Speech Pathologist

Speech pathologists have different approaches and styles. They also have techniques they prefer to use. Before parents commit to working with a speech pathologist, it would be beneficial to ask her some basic questions. These would be:

✓ "Will you or someone else be working with my child?" Some private practices employ a few speech pathologists. Parents will want to talk directly with the person who will work with their child when they ask the questions.

✓ "What is your experience working with preschoolers who stutter?"

✓ "What approach do you use when working with preschoolers?"

✓ "How successful has your approach been?"

✓ "What would be a short term goal?"

✓ "How long do you feel it would take to meet that goal?"

✓ "How are parents involved in therapy?"

✓ "Will my child have homework?"

✓ "What should we expect from therapy?"

✓ "How long do you anticipate therapy will take?"

✓ "Is there anything else I should know before starting therapy?"

Parents may want to speak with two or three speech pathologists before selecting the one to work with their child.

Getting Therapy To Work For The Child

Once parents have selected a speech pathologist, it is critical that they be consistent in bringing their child in for his scheduled appointments. Also, once a speech pathologist has been selected to work with the child, it is important that the child work with her until the child has completed therapy. Inconsistency can thwart the best efforts of any speech pathologist working with a child. Starting and stopping therapy, and/or switching speech pathologists can be ingredients for stuttering therapy failure.

How often will the child need therapy? I require that parents commit to no fewer than twice weekly, thirty minute therapy sessions of individual therapy each week in order for a child to progress. Less than that and progress will either become frustratingly slow or there will be no changes. I reduce to once a week therapy after that child has remained fluent for two to three weeks, once every two weeks for continued fluency, and then dismissal from therapy.

Fluency therapy for the preschool child can be completed in a relatively short period of time with the cooperation of the parents. Improvements should be noticed within the first three months of beginning therapy. If the child has not improved noticeably by the three month point, it is time to for the parents and the therapist to meet to discuss why no improvement has occurred. Parents can ask the child's therapist to give a timeframe within which improvement should occur. Below is a list that highlights possible reasons for lack of sufficient progress in therapy. It is also shown as Chart Three on p. 95. If there is no reasonable explanation for lack of progress, parents may want to seek the opinion of another speech pathologist.

Problem: Parents are not involved in therapy.

Why Counterproductive: Parents and therapist are not working together for the benefit of the child.

Solution: Parents should ask the therapist how they can help. The therapist should offer suggestions to the parents.

Problem: Therapy is inconsistent.

Why Counterproductive: Consistency is vital to progress. Lack of consistency can slow progress down or bring it to a halt. This can frustrate all involved and make it appear as if therapy does not help.

Solution: Children should attend all scheduled sessions.

Problem: Therapy does not occur frequently enough.

Why Counterproductive: Therapy less than twice weekly is inadequate because young children quickly forget what they learned unless it is reinforced in a reasonable amount of time. If progress is too slow, everyone loses interest in therapy.

Solution: Therapy should take place no less than twice weekly, until the child has achieved fluency.

Problem: The child is in group therapy.

Why Counterproductive: Individual attention to a child and his speech issue is reduced when the therapist's attention is divided among other children.

Solution: Place the child in individual therapy.

Problem: The child changes therapists.

Why Counterproductive: It is important for the child to bond with the therapist. Switching therapists means that the child has to form a new bond and adjust to a different person and therapy style. (Sometimes changing therapists is in the best interest of the child. Parents should be careful not to make it a pattern.)

Solution: Talk to the therapist about her program before you commit.

Problem: The child works with two therapists.

Why Counterproductive: The different therapy styles and treatment methods can confuse the child.

Solution: Sometimes a child is seen for therapy by the school speech pathologist and the parents want to supplement therapy privately. Select one speech pathologist to work on fluency with the child.

Problem: Frequent therapy breaks.

Why Counterproductive: Therapy breaks are disruptive to the therapeutic process. Until the child has achieved fluency, breaks can result in relapse.

Solution: Parents should maintain the therapy schedule. If the child will not attend therapy for a week or two, parents should ask the therapist what they can do so that regression does not occur. If summer vacation is approaching and the parents will not be able to commit to consistent therapy, it is best to wait until the break ends before starting therapy.

In my experience, the problems listed above can make therapy counterproductive. Once therapy becomes counter-productive, parents may feel that therapy does not work. The child, as he gets older, may also believe that therapy is of no use.

Chapter Recap

✓ There are numerous markers that indicate when seeking professional therapy may be necessary.

✓ Seek out therapists who are licensed and or certified and have had experience working with young children who stutter.

✓ Speech pathologists work in private practices and public school districts.

✓ The speech pathologist will ask the parent(s) numerous questions about the child's speech history.

✓ The speech pathologist will work closely with the family.

✓ The speech pathologist will tailor a therapy program for the child.

✓ There can be various reasons for lack of progress in therapy.

Chapter Six

Questions and Answers

Common Concerns and Questions

When Did Adults Who Stutter Begin Stuttering?

Stuttering begins to take root in the preschool years. Most adults who stutter began stuttering sometime before their fifth birthday.

Is My Child's Disfluency Permanent?

I would like to start out with a word of reassurance. Disfluent speech, during the preschool years, is so common that I would say it is a normal occurrence. The odds are in your child's favor that the disfluency is temporary. Stuttering need not be permanent. However, what you do can determine how quickly your child gains control of his speech.

Is My Child Aware of His Disfluencies?

Most children are aware of changes in their speech although they may not talk about it. As a matter of fact, older children may deny that they stutter even though many have already consciously begun to avoid stuttering.

Is My Child Stuttering On Purpose to Get Attention?

Absolutely not. Children do not use stuttering as an attention getting behavior. However, it may be that your child stutters more when he is trying to get someone's attention. That is because your child may feel frustrated trying to get your

attention and frustration can result in an increase
in disfluencies.

Does It Mean My Child Has Emotional Problems Because He Stutters?

Stuttering is not an indicator of emotional problems. However, strong emotions can result in an increase in disfluencies. If you feel there are issues that are causing your child to suffer emotionally, it is best to get those issues resolved.

Is My Child Bothered By His Disfluencies?

Some preschoolers are bothered by it, others are not. It probably depends on the degree to which it occurs, and the child's ability to communicate effectively and the reaction of others to his speech. If your child is bothered by his disfluencies, he may not necessarily tell you. Indicators that your child may be bothered by his speech are:

- ✓ He may avoid talking.
- ✓ He may look to you to talk for him.
- ✓ He may show frustration when talking.
- ✓ He may get angry or throw temper tantrums.
- ✓ He may hit, bite or kick other children.
- ✓ He may choose to play by himself rather than interact with other children.
- ✓ His teacher may say that he rarely talks in class.

What Conditions Can Affect My Child's Fluency?

You may have noticed that your child's speech is fluent under certain conditions. Given other conditions, your child may become disfluent. Each child is different. Your child's speaking environment, the behavior and attitude of the listener, and his emotions when talking, can individually, or together, affect his fluency.

Why Does My Child Go Through Periods of No Stuttering?

Adults who stutter also experience brief periods of fluency only to find that they start stuttering again. Preschool children experience this as well. Sometimes those periods of no stuttering are unexplainable. Generally, however, your child will be more fluent when he is feeling at ease and comfortable. Try to find a pattern between his fluent periods and his environment.

Why Doesn't My Child Stutter When He Talks to Our Baby or Dog?

Babies and animals are uncritical listeners and give unconditional love. This can be comforting for a child who stutters and puts him at ease. The result is that the child speaks fluently.

Have I Done Something to Cause the "Stuttering?"

No. Disfluent speech, in preschoolers, is a normal and common occurrence. However, it is important to be aware of the do's and don'ts of helping your child.

Should I Wait to Do Anything About My Child's Repetitions And Hesitations?

Do not wait. Begin to make the positive changes described in this book. Know when the child needs to see a speech pathologist.

Does Stress or Anxiety Cause Stuttering?

It is not known what causes stuttering but stress and anxiety do not cause it. However, stress and anxiety can contribute to the severity of the stutter. A person who stutters may find it more difficult to control a stutter when he is stressed.

What Should I Do If I See Secondary Behaviors?

Secondary stuttering behaviors are body or facial movements show up after a child has been disfluent for a few months. In his struggle to speak, a child may blink his eyes, move his eyeballs sideways, raise his upper lip, tilt his head, jerk his head or have visible lip, facial or jaw tension. These are just a few examples of non-speech behaviors. There are others.

It is best to ignore secondary behaviors. Listen to what the child is saying not how he is saying it. However, the arrival of secondary behaviors may mean that it is time to seek the help of a professional.

Is It Better to Do Speech Therapy in a Small Group Setting or Individually?

It is best to do speech therapy individually. In individual therapy, the speech pathologist will give the child her undivided attention. However, small group settings for older children and adults can offer support and encouragement.

How Does Having a Calmer Home Life Help My Child's Stutter?

Environments that induce anxiety, stress, and other strong emotions can contribute to stuttering. A calm environment would tend to offer fewer occasions for strong emotional reactions. That does not mean that a child will cease to stutter in a calm environment. It may, however, reduce the emotional catalysts that contribute to stuttering.

I Feel That My Speech Therapist Is Not Helping My Child. I Feel Guilty Switching Therapists. How Can I Change Therapists Without Hurting Her Feelings?

I think many people can relate to this concern, whether it be changing doctors, hairdressers or speech pathologists. Before switching, I would talk to the speech pathologist. Ask her questions about your child's therapy that have caused you to think about switching. Some possible questions would be:

✓ How do you feel about my child's progress so far?

✓ How long do you anticipate therapy will take?

✓ What are the short term goals and how long do you feel it will take to reach them?

✓ Do you feel there is something standing in the way of my child's progress?

Her answers may help you decide to give therapy with her a bit more time or convince you to switch. In the event you decide to switch, keep in mind that you need to do what is best for your child regardless of the feelings of the professional. If that time comes, here are a couple of suggestions:

✓ Tell her that you are concerned about your child's progress. You understand that each professional has different approaches to stuttering therapy and you have decided that another approach may be more effective with your child. Tell her you appreciate what she has done up until now.

✓ If you are close to summer or winter break, ask the speech pathologist to cancel your child's appointments for now. Parents often use those times to make changes in their child's schedule.

Professionals understand that clients make changes as they see fit and that they need to do what they feel is in their child's best interests. Remember, concern about hurting the feelings of a professional becomes irrelevant when it comes to doing what is best for one's child.

How Do I Find a Good Therapist?

The American Speech-Language and Hearing Association has a list of certified speech pathologists in each state on their website

at www.asha.org. Once you navigate to that site, read the
areas of specialty that the speech pathologists feel comfortable
treating. Speech pathologists who feel stuttering is their area
of expertise will state so. The American Speech-Language
Association and the Stuttering Foundation have the names of
speech pathologists, in your state, who work with individuals
who stutter. The ASHA website for finding a professional near
you is http://www.asha.org/findpro. The Stuttering Foundation
website is http://www.stutteringhelp. org/referrals-information.

How Long Will It Take Before I See Improvements?

The answer to this question hinges on factors such as the
parents' diligence and consistency in bringing their child to the
therapy sessions, parental follow through on the suggestions
made by the speech pathologist, if the child is in individual or
group sessions, the number of sessions the child is seen per week,
the amount of time the child spends in each session and the
severity of the child's stutter.

The best case scenario is individual therapy sessions two
to three times per week for thirty minutes each session. The
parents are consistent in bringing their child to the sessions and
are diligent in following through on the therapist's suggestions.
With these contingencies in place, it should take three to six
months to see improvement in the preschool child's speech.

What Should I Do If My Child Is Older And Has Started Stuttering?

I would seek out the help of a speech pathologist. The sooner
you seek out professional help for a child older than five
the better.

Are There Sounds and Words Children Will Stutter More On?

There are no specific sounds or words that cause children to
stutter. However, as the child struggles with his speech he may

try to figure out why he is stuttering. If he stutters a few times on, let us say, the "s" sound, he may assume that the sound causes him to stutter. He may avoid saying words that start with that sound. Or he may say, "I can't say that sound."

Why Would I Pay for Therapy If It Is Free in the Public Schools?

The difference between private services and public services is more than money. It is also the manner in which services are provided. Getting therapy for your child in the public schools is a process. First, you must contact the public schools and tell them about your child's problem. They will want your child to be screened by a speech pathologist in the district. Once your child is screened, a decision will be made whether your child's problem is severe enough to warrant testing or if your child should be rescreened next year. If the decision is made to test, your child must be tested within a specified amount of time following the screening. If the testing finds that your child is not eligible for services, you will be asked to wait until next year. If your child's speech meets the criteria for eligibility for services, the professional will write your child's goals for the year in an Individualized Education Plan (IEP). This entire process can take three months or more.

Public school services run on a school calendar year. When school is not in session, your child will not have speech therapy. This interrupts progress. Your child may be fortunate to have a half-hour of individual therapy. As a rule though, therapy is provided to small groups of two to five children of different ages with different speech problems. The sessions are a half-hour for all children in the group. You can determine how many minutes of therapy your child gets by dividing 30 minutes by the number of children in the room. Thus, two children would get 15 minutes of therapy each, three children 10 minutes and so on. Perhaps your child's therapist schedules two half-hour sessions for your child each week. All too common is the once weekly therapy session. The public school's speech pathologist is the one your child will work with; parents have no choice in the matter.

If you decide to seek therapy with a speech pathologist in private practice, you can select someone who is experienced working with preschool children who stutter. The evaluation should take no more than an hour. The decision to start therapy can be made then or on the subsequent visit. You will see the professional each time you bring your child in for therapy and you can ask about the child's progress during the session. With private therapy, your child will be seen individually for the entire session. Therapy will be more consistent because private therapy does not run according to the school calendar. Therapy is year round and can be scheduled for two or three sessions a week. This allows for greater consistency in therapy and faster progress.

Once you have committed to therapy, it is important to make it a priority. It should be more important than sports, dancing lessons, music lessons, etc. There are good speech pathologist in the public schools and in private practice. I know how appealing free can be. But consider that free services can cost more in the long run if the problem is not treated in a timely fashion. This is your child's future and that should be the priority.

Will Learning Another Language
Cause My Child to Stutter or Stutter More?

There is no evidence that learning a second language will cause a child to stutter or stutter more. If the child is bilingual, the parents should avoid mixing words from both languages in the same sentence when speaking with him. However, the child should be allowed to mix words from both language when he speaks.

Will My Health Insurance Cover for Speech Services?

It is worthwhile to review one's policy or contact a health insurance representative to ask about their coverage for speech services. Ask the health insurance representative if they cover for *evaluation of speech fluency* and therapy for *childhood onset fluency disorder*. They may want codes for these services. The CPT code for *evaluation of speech fluency* is 92521 and the diagnostic code for *childhood onset fluency disorder* is 315.35. If one's health insurance does provide coverage, it is important for the parent to ask the representative to specify the limits of coverage. Some health plans cover for the evaluation and therapy, others for only the evaluation, others for only therapy, there may be monetary caps and so on.

How Much Does Private Speech Therapy Cost?

The cost of private therapy can be costly and the price varies within cities and states. I suggest that parents think of it as an investment in the child's future the cost of which will only go up as the child gets older. This is because waiting beyond the preschool years means therapy will take longer. As children get habituated to their speech pattern, the longer it will take for therapy to change it. Thus, it is important to consider therapy a financial priority.

Information Records

Please use this information record to help organize observations and information. If seeking professional help, this checklist will assist the speech pathologist in better understanding the child's problem. In two parent households, since parents may have different perceptions of the problems, each parent should answer the questions independently of the other.

My child began stuttering when he/she was _____ years old.

The first person who noticed the stutter was

_____.

Is there a family member who stutters?

Do you feel that something caused the stuttering? Describe below:

How do you feel your child feels about his/her stuttering?

        Frustrated____
        Refuses to talk__
        Embarrassed____
        Angry____
        Doesn't seem to care____

Does your child do any of the following:

         Avoids certain words___

         Changes words___

         Avoids talking___

         Loses his/her temper___

         Hits other children___

Does any of the following happen when your child is trying to get his/her words out:

         Eyes blink___

         Eyes move sideways___

         Lips quiver___

         Inhales deeply___

         Body stiffens___

         Head jerks___

         Stamps foot___

         Other secondary characteristics_____

         _____

My child's speech is better

         In the morning__

         After school___

         At night___

         When talking to a pet___

         When talking to (name of the person(s)

         _____

         When relaxed___

         When playing with_____

         When reciting (numbers, nursery rhyme, alphabet)

         _____

         When singing___

My child's speech is worse

         In the morning__

         After school___

         At night___

         When talking to (name of the person(s))

         _____

         When playing with_____

When tired___
When hungry___
When frustrated___
When angry___
When anxious___
When stressed___
When excited___
When afraid___
What has been said or done to help the child stop stuttering?

How concerned are you about your child's speech?
    Not concerned at all___
    Somewhat concerned___
    Very concerned___
    Extremely concerned___
How well does the child get along with:
    Mother
    Father
    Brother(s)

    Sister(s)

What does the child enjoy doing?

What does the child dislike doing?

Chart One: Dos and Don'ts

Avoid Saying or Doing	Reason	Instead Say or Do
"Say it again," "Say it again this way," or "Say it the way I say it."	You do not want the child to feel that how he talks is wrong or that he is bad because he is disfluent. Also, saying it again does not insure that the next time will be better.	Listen to what your child is saying. Respond to what he said, not how he said it.
"Speak slower," "Slow down," or "You are talking too fast."*	The child's speaking rate is not going to determine whether or not he will stutter.	Listen to what your child is saying. Respond to what he said, not how he said it. Focusing on rate of speech will not eliminate a stutter. The child, if he knows what you mean by slowing down, will simply speak slower and stutter. The child will need to learn to control his speech. As he struggles with his speech, he may discover that slower speech allows him greater control over how he speaks. As he learns control, he may slow his rate on his own.
"Think before you speak" or "Think about how you are talking."	Thinking before speaking will not eliminate a stutter. Should the child think about what he wants to say or how it should come out?	Listen to what your child is saying. Respond to what he said, not how he said it.

Chart One: Dos and Don'ts (Continued)

Avoid Saying or Doing	Reason	Instead Say or Do
"I am not going to listen to you if you talk that way."	It is extremely important that the child feels that what he has to say is important. It is important for a child's self-concept and his desire to improve his communication skills. Refusing to listen to a child because he stutters can convey the idea that what he has to say is not important unless his speech meets a fluency standard. What a child has to say is important no matter how it is said.	Listen to what your child is saying. Respond to what he said, not how he said it.
"Every time you talk that way you will get punished."	If a child is disfluent, he has not figured out how to control this aspect of his speech. If he cannot yet control his disfluent speech, but he can control whether or not he speaks, your child may avoid speaking in order to avoid a punishment. Speech avoidance is not uncommon among children for whom stuttering has been a problem. You do not want your child to avoid speaking since that can lead to other issues.	Listen to what your child is saying. Respond to what he said, not how he said it.
"Calm down." "Relax before you talk."*	Children do not stutter because they are not calm or relaxed. True, stuttering can increase when a child feels a strong emotion. But strong emotions contribute to, rather than cause, the problem. Important are the reasons for the strong emotions. Advising the child to calm down or relax before talking focuses attention on the stuttering without discovering the cause of the strong emotions. There have been children who have told me that such advice made them so angry, they stuttered more as a result.	Listen to what your child is saying. Respond to what he said, not how he said it.

"Take a deep breath before you talk."	By saying this you are suggesting to the young child that deep breathing before talking helps him to avoid stuttering. Untrue. A deep breath before talking may distract the child the first couple of times resulting in a fluent start. However you may find that the child takes a deep breath and stutters anyhow. There is also the risk that the instruction may lead to a block. The child may take a deep breath, hold it and then push out the word. Or, it may become a secondary stuttering characteristic. In other words, the child may begin to believe that he cannot talk fluently without taking a deep breath. As a result, he may take a deep breath before he says anything, becoming an attention grabbing behavior on its own.**	Listen to what your child is saying. Respond to what he said, not how he said it. Avoid giving him advice.
"Stop talking that way."	Since children and adults do not stutter on purpose, it is not helpful to tell them to stop.	Listen to what your child is saying. Respond to what he said, not how he said it.
Speaking for your child or finishing words or sentences no matter how strong the urge.	This can be very frustrating for the child.	Listen to what your child is saying until he is done. Then respond to what he has said.
Interrupting your child when he is speaking.	Interrupting the child is disruptive and can be frustrating. It was found that parents of children who stutter interrupt their children more often than do parents of children who do not stutter (Kasprisin-Burrelli, et al).	Listen to what your child is saying until he is done. Then respond to what he has said.***

Chart One: Dos and Don'ts (Continued)

Avoid Saying or Doing	Reason	Instead Say or Do
Speaking for your child to help him or because you are embarrassed by his speech or you believe he is.	Children can sense when their parents feel bad or are embarrassed by what they are doing. Your child may feel worse about his speech if he senses your discomfort.	Allow your child to speak and complete his thoughts on his own. Do not help him or speak for him.
Facial or body language shows that you are anxious or upset when your child is talking.	Sometimes facial expressions can convey as much information as words.	Listen calmly and patiently to your child. Make sure that your facial expression does not convey a negative emotion about how he is talking.
Asking your child to perform or recite in front of other people.	There are children who dislike performing on the spot.	Proudly tell others what your child can do without asking him to perform or recite.
Talking about your child's speech to other people while he is present.	The child may be embarrassed that you are talking about him. The exception is if you are talking with the speech pathologist who will work with your child.	Speak to the other person at a time when the child is not present.
Getting upset or distressed when your child is disfluent.	Seeing a parent distressed or upset because he has stuttered can make a child feel bad.	Listen unemotionally to how your child has spoken. Express your emotions to what he has said rather than how he has said it.
Calling your child a "stutterer."	Stuttering is something the child does, not who he is. This period in your child's life does not define him.	Accept your child as he is without labeling him.

Limiting the amount of time your child has to speak.	Time pressure can result in an increase in stuttering.	Allow your child to say what he would like to say no matter how long it takes.
Bombarding your child with questions.	It can be overwhelming for anyone to respond to many questions at once.	Calmly ask your child a question and patiently wait for the answer. Keep questions short and simple. Respond to what your child has said before you ask another question.
Poking fun of your child's speech by imitating or teasing him.	This behavior can result in a range of emotions. The child may avoid talking.	Listen to what your child has said without commenting on how he has spoken.

* Rapid speech and strong emotional reactions are issues that should be dealt with on their own and not in relation to stuttering, at this point. If the help of a speech pathologist is sought, she will consider these issues as she plans a therapy program.

** I worked with a preschool boy who stuttered moderately. He was making nice progress in therapy. One weekend his parents went out of town and his grandparents came into town to take care of him and his sister. When he came to our first therapy session, after that weekend, he could barely speak. He continually gulped for air as he tried to speak. It was a wonder he did not hyperventilate. During our session, I was able to learn from him what had happened. To "help" him stop stuttering, his grandparents had instructed him to "breathe" before he talked.

*** When a child who stutters is interrupted or interrupts another person, he usually stutters more than if there is no interruption. A study was done to determine how conversational turn-taking affected the speech of a five-year-old boy who stuttered. The results of the study showed that when conversational turn-taking was instituted, the five-year-old's stuttering decreased. When the turn-taking rule was ignored the child stuttered more (Winslow).

Chart Two: What to Look for in the Child's Preschool

Negative Attributes	Positive Attributes
The environment is noisy.	Children and adults use their "indoor" voices. If music is playing, its volume is low.
Children are walking or running around aimlessly.	Children are engaged in activities and the adults are engaged with them.
You observe children pushing, pulling, hitting or kicking other children or teachers.	Children are respectful of one another and "use their words" instead of resorting to negative physical contact.
Children are sitting around with nothing to do.	Children are playing or talking with one another.
There are too few adults in the room for the number of children.	The ratio varies with the age of the children. There should be fewer children per adult for younger children. Check your state's guidelines.
There are a lot of people in the room. Overcrowding is a problem.	The room is large enough to accommodate the number of people in it.
The caregivers are inattentive to the children and their needs.	The caregivers are focused on the children and engaged with them.
The caregivers look grumpy or frazzled.	The caregivers should look happy.
The teachers use criticism when talking to the children.	Teachers should use positive words and be generous with praise. When a child has done something wrong, the teacher should ask the child to say what he has done that was wrong. The teacher should ask him how he could have handled the problem differently and assist him as needed.
Teachers swap classrooms during the day reducing the children's consistency with caregivers.	The children have the same teachers throughout the day, every day.
The school has a high teacher turnover rate.	The school retains the same teachers throughout the year.
Children tease one another.	Children are respectful of the other children.

Chart Three: Getting Therapy to Work for the Child

Problem	Why Counterproductive	Solution
Parents are not involved in therapy.	Parents and therapist are not working together for the benefit of the child.	Parents should ask the therapist how they can help. The therapist should offer suggestions to the parents.
Therapy is inconsistent.	Consistency is vital to progress. Lack of consistency can slow progress down or bring it to a halt. This can frustrate all involved and make it appear as if therapy does not help.	Children should attend all scheduled sessions.
Therapy does not occur frequently enough.	Therapy less than twice weekly is inadequate because young children quickly forget what they learned unless it is reinforced in a reasonable amount of time. If progress is too slow, everyone loses interest in therapy.	Therapy should take place no less than twice weekly, until the child has achieved fluency.
The child is in group therapy.	Individual attention to a child and his speech issue is reduced when the therapist's attention is divided among other children.	Place the child in individual therapy.

Getting Therapy to Work for the Child (Continued)

Problem	Why Counterproductive	Solution
The child changes therapists.	It is important for the child to bond with the therapist. Switching therapists means that the child has to form a new bond and adjust to a different person and therapy style. (Sometimes changing therapists is in the best interest of the child. Parents should be careful not to make it a pattern.)	Talk to the therapist about her program before you commit.
The child works with two therapists.	The different therapy styles and treatment methods can confuse the child.	Sometimes a child is seen for therapy by the school speech pathologist and the parents want to supplement therapy privately. Select one speech pathologist to work on fluency with the child.

| Frequent therapy breaks. | Therapy breaks are disruptive to the therapeutic process. Until the child has achieved fluency, breaks can result in relapse. | Parents should maintain the therapy schedule. If the child will not attend therapy for a week or two, parents should ask the therapist what they can do so that regression does not occur. If summer vacation is approaching and the parents will not be able to commit to consistent therapy, it is best to wait until the break ends before starting therapy. |

Table 1:	PHYSICIAN'S CHECKLIST FOR REFERRAL		
	The Child With NORMAL DISFLUENCIES Age of Onset: 1½ to 7 years of age	The Child With MILD STUTTERING Age of Onset: 1½ to 7 years of age	The Child With SEVERE STUTTERING Age of Onset: 1½ to 7 years of age
Speech behavior you may see or hear:	☐ Occasional (not more than once in every 10 sentences), brief, (typical ½ second or shorter) repetitions of sounds, syllables or short words, e.g., li-li-like this.	☐ Frequent (3% or more of speech), long (½ to 1 second) repetitions of sounds, syllables, or short words, e.g., li-li-li-like this. Occasional prolongations of sounds.	☐ Very frequent (10% or more of speech), and often very long (1 second or longer) repetitions of sounds, syllables or short words. Frequent sound prolongations and blockages.
Other behavior you may see or hear:	☐ Occasional pauses, hesitations in speech or fillers such as "uh," "er," or "um," changing of words or thoughts.	☐ Repetitions and prolongations begin to be associated with eyelid closing and blinking, looking to the side, and some physical tension in and around the lips.	☐ Similar to mild stutterers only more frequent and noticeable; some rise in pitch of voice during stuttering. Extra sounds or words used as "starters."

When problems most noticeable:	☐ Tends to come and go when child is: tired, excited, talking about complex/new topics, asking or answering questions or talking to unresponsive listeners.	☐ Tends to come and go in similar situations, but is more often present than absent.	☐ Tends to be present in most speaking situations; far more consistent and non-fluctuating.
Child reaction:	☐ None apparent	☐ Some show little concern, some will be frustrated and embarrassed.	☐ Most are embarrassed and some are also fearful of speaking.
Parent reaction:	☐ None to a great deal	☐ Most concerned, but concern may be minimal.	☐ All have some degree of concern.
Referral decision:	☐ Refer only if parents moderately to overly concerned.	☐ Refer if continues for 6 to 8 weeks or if parental concern justifies it.	☐ Refer as soon as possible.

Further Reading

For more information on stuttering, the Speech Foundation offers information and a series of excellent books, ebooks, brochures and videos on stuttering. Their website is www.stutteringhelp.org. The National Stuttering Association offers support to individuals who stutter and their families. Their website is www.nsastutter.org. The website for the International Stuttering Association is: www.isastutter.org.

Books On Stuttering

- ✓ *Understanding Stammering or Stuttering: A Guide for Parents, Teachers and Other Professionals* by Elaine Kelman and Alison Whyte, (2012).

- ✓ *Stuttering in Preschool Age* by Zbigniew Tarkowski, Ewa Humeniuk and Jolanta Dunaj.

- ✓ *Hooray for Aiden* by Karen Hollett. This the story of how Aiden, a young girl who stutters, overcomes her fear of speaking in front of classmates at her new school. This book is appropriate for children ages 4-9.

- ✓ *If Your Child Stutters: A Guide for Parents* by Stanley Ainsworth, Ph.D. and Jane Fraser.

- ✓ *Notes to the Teacher: The Child Who Stutters at Schools* by Lisa Scott. This is an informative brochure offered by the Stuttering Foundation advises teachers in how to assist children who stutter.

- ✓ *Why Speech Therapy?* This Stuttering Foundation brochure covers topics such as why seek out speech therapy, the amount, length and cost, expectations for success, therapy goals and selecting a speech pathologist.

✓ *Stuttering and Your Child: Help for Parents* by Richard F. Curlee, Edward G. Conture. Available as a DVD or book, the focus is to help families understand stuttering and make changes to promote more fluent speech.

✓ *The Child Who Stutters: To the Pediatrician* by Barry Guitar, and Edward G. Conture. Stuttering Foundation free downloadable book found at http://www.stutteringhelp. org/free-e-books

✓ *Stuttering: Straight Talk for Teachers* by Lisa Scott. Stuttering Foundation free downloadable book found at http://www.stutteringhelp.org/free-e-books

✓ *Young Children Who Stutter Ages 2-6* by J. Scott Yaruss, PhD, & Nina Reardon, MA. This book gives information about stuttering and, in particular, young children who stutter.

✓ *Special Education and the Law* by Lisa Scott. This brochure is available at the Stuttering Foundation's website.

Bibliography

Beilby, J., Byrnes, M., Young K. (2012). The experiences of living with a sibling who stutters: A preliminary study. *Journal of Fluency Disorders*, 37, 135–148.

Beitchman, J.H., et al (1994). Seven-year follow-up of speech/language-impaired and control children: speech/language stability and outcome. *Journal of the American Academy of Child Adolescent Psychiatry*, 33, 1322–1330.

Chang, Soo-Eun , Erickson Kirk I., Ambrose, Nicoline G. , Hasegawa-Johnson, Mark A. , & Ludlow, Christy L. (2008). Brain Anatomy Differences in Childhood Stuttering. *Neuroimaging*, 39, 1333–1344.

Conture, E., Choi, D. Jones, R. (2013). Temperament, Stuttering and Their Possible Association. National Stuttering Association Presentation.

Cooper, E. (1993). Chronic perseverative stuttering syndrome: a harmful or helpful construct. *American Journal of Speech-Language Pathology*, 2, 11–15.

De Nil, L. & Brutten, G. (1991). Speech-associated attitudes of stuttering and nonstuttering children. *Journal of Speech and Hearing Research*, 34, 60–66.

Guitar, B., Kopff Shaefer, H., Donahue-Kilburg, G., and Bond, L. (1992). Parent Verbal Interactions and Speech Rate: A Case Study in Stuttering. *Journal of Speech and Hearing Research*, 35, 742–754.

Kalinowski, J., Stuart, A., & Armson, J. (1996). Perceptions of stutterers and nonstutterers during speaking and nonspeaking situations. *American Journal of Speech-Language Pathology*, 5, 61-66.

Kasprisin-Burrelli, A., Egolf, D., & Shames, G. (1972). A comparison of parental verbal behavior with stuttering and nonstuttering children. *Journal of Communication Disorders*, 5, 335–346.

Lass, N.J., et al. (1992). Teachers' perceptions of stutterers. *Language Speech and Hearing Services in Schools*, 23, 78–81.

Lass, N.J., et al. (1994). School administrators' perceptions of people who stutter. *Language Speech and Hearing Services in Schools*, 25, 90–93.

Miles, S. & Ratner, N.B. (2001). Parental Language Input to Children at Stuttering Onset. J Speech Lang Hear Research, 44, 1116–1130.

Ramig, P.R. (1993). High reported spontaneous stuttering recovery rates: fact or fiction? *Language Speech and Hearing Services in Schools*, 24, 156–160.

Starkweather, C.W. & Gottwald S.R. (1993). A pilot study of relations among specific measures obtained at intake and discharge in a program of prevention and early intervention for stuttering. *American Journal of Speech-Language Pathology*, 2, 51–58.

Winslow, M. & Guitar, B. (1994). The effects of structured turn-taking on disfluencies. *Language, Speech, and Hearing Services in Schools*, 25, 251–257.

Yairi, E., (1993). Epidemiologic and other considerations in treatment efficacy research with preschool age children who stutter. *Journal of Fluency Disorders*, 18, 197–219.

Yairi, E., & Ambrose, N. (1992). Onset of stuttering in preschool children: selected factors. *Journal of Speech and Hearing Research*, 35, 782–788.

Yairi, E. & Carrico, D. (1992). Early childhood stuttering: pediatricians' attitudes and practices. *American Journal of Speech-Language Pathology*, 1, 54–62.

Zackheim, C., & Conture, E. (2003). Childhood stuttering and speech disfluencies in relation to children's mean length of utterance: A preliminary study. *Journal of Fluency Disorders*, 28, 115–142

Zebrowski, P. & Schum, R. (1993). Counseling parents of children who stutter. *American Journal of Speech-Language Pathology*, 2, 65–73.

Index

Note: a *c* indicates a chart; a *t*, a table.

F

Facial expressions, 25, 92c
Facts about, 6–7
FAPE. *See* Free appropriate public
  education
Fatigue, effect of on fluency, 51
Fears, 32–33
Financial problems, effect of on
  fluency, 53
Finishing words and sentences, 24,
  91c
Fluency
    periodic, 77
    and uncritical listeners, 77
Forms of stuttering, 12
Free appropriate public education
  (FAPE), 64
Frequency of therapy, 71, 95c
Frustration, 28–29
Frustration caused by advice, 20

G

Gender and frequency of stuttering,
  3, 4
Group therapy, 72, 78, 95c
Guilt, 18–19

H

Habituation of speech patterns, 67
Helping child, 20–21
Helping others help child
    other children, 59
    relatives and adult friends, 58
    siblings, 55–57
    teachers and daycare givers,
      57–58
Home environment
    balanced/calm environment,
      42–43, 78
    chaotic environment, 41
    hostile environment, 42
    Ordinary Magic, 40

perfectionistic/strict
  environment, 41–42
quality of child-parent
  relationships, 39–40
Hostile home environment, 42

I

IDEA. *See* Individuals with
  Disabilities Act, Amendments of
  1997
Ignoring, 22, 90c
Illness, effect of on fluency, 51, 52–53
Impact of stuttering, 11
Individuals with Disabilities Act,
  Amendments of 1997 (IDEA), 64
Individual therapy versus group
  therapy, 78
Information records, 85–87
Insurance coverage
    childhood onset fluency
      disorder diagnosis, 67, 83
    evaluation of speech fluency
      provision, 67, 83
    neurological basis
      requirement, 68
Interrupting, 24, 91c
Interrupting, stopping, home
  environment, 44–45

L

Labeling, 26, 92c
Licensure, 63
Limiting time to speak, 27, 93c
Listening, 33–34
Listening skills, 34
Love, expressing, 47

M

Mild stutter, 14
Moderate stutter, 14
Monster Study, 11
Multiple therapists, 72, 96c

Acknowledgments

I would like to thank Sandy Lieberman, Ellen Douglass, Pattie Wood, Mary Macuga, and Susan Wildman for sharing their insights and opinions. I would like to also thank Steve Wildman for his help in arriving at the title of this book.

I would like to thank my husband, Zohar Raz, for his support and technical knowledge.

Notes

How to Teach a Child to Say the "R" Sound in 15 Easy Lessons

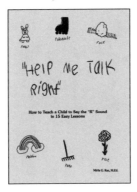

This "Help Me Talk Right" book focuses on the "r" sound. It presents an easy to follow, proven step-by-step method of correcting those pesky "r"s. All the tools and techniques you need for "r" sound correction are included.

Free of technical jargon and easy to use, this book is for speech pathologists, speech assistants, and parents who wish to teach a child how to say the "r" sound and use it in conversation. Everything you need to know about teaching a child to say and use the "r" sound is clearly shown in a step-by-step format. Each lesson builds upon the successes of previous lessons so that the child is challenged to use the "r" more often until she is able to use it in conversation. The book comes complete with worksheets, suggestions for games and fun exercises, and a certificate of achievement.

Contents

Prelesson
One: Tongue and Teeth Positioning
Two: Producing the RRRRR Sound
Three: Final RRRRR in Simple Syllables
Four: Initial RRRRR in Simple Syllables
Five: Final RRRRR in Simple Words
Six: Initial RRRRR in Simple Words
Seven: Pairing Initial RRRRR Simple Words
Eight: Pairing Final RRRRR Simple Words
Nine: Medial RRRRR in Simple Words
Ten: Final RRRRR in Simple Sentences
Eleven: Initial RRRRR in Simple Sentences
Twelve: Blends
Thirteen: Sentences Using Initial, Medial, and Final RRRRR and RRRRR in Blends
Fourteen: Using RRRRR While Playing
Fifteen: Using RRRRR in Conversation
Certificate of Achievement
Appendix A: Worksheets
Appendix B: Activities & Materials

Orders and information:
GerstenWeitz Publishers
8356 E. San Rafael Dr.
Scottsdale, AZ 85258
Phone: (480) 951-9707   Fax: (480) 993-2169
E-mail: info@speechbooks.com
www.helpmetalkright.com

How to Teach a Child to Say the "L" Sound in 15 Easy Lessons

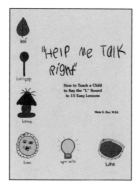

This "Help Me Talk Right" book focuses on the "l" sound. It presents an easy to follow, proven step-by-step method of correcting those funny sounding 'l's. All the tools and techniques you need for "l" sound correction are included.

Free of technical jargon and easy to use, this book is for speech pathologists, speech assistants, and parents who wish to teach a child how to say the "l" sound and use it in conversation. Everything you need to know about teaching a child to say and use the "l" sound is clearly shown in a step-by-step format. Each lesson builds upon the successes of previous lessons so that the child is challenged to use the "l" more often until he is able to use it in conversation. The book comes complete with worksheets, suggestions for games and fun exercises, and a certificate of achievement.

Contents

Prelesson
One: Tongue Positioning
Two: Producing the LLLLL Sound
Three: Initial LLLLL in Simple Syllables
Four: Final LLLLL in Simple Syllables
Five: Initial LLLLL in Simple Words
Six: Final LLLLL in Simple Words
Seven: Pairing Initial LLLLL Simple Words
Eight: Pairing Final LLLLL Simple Words
Nine: Medial LLLLL in Simple Words
Ten: Initial LLLLL in Simple Sentences
Eleven: Final LLLLL in Simple Sentences
Twelve: LLLLL in Blends
Thirteen: Sentences Using Initial, Medial, and Final LLLLL and LLLLL in Blends
Fourteen: Using LLLLL While Playing
Fifteen: Using LLLLL in Conversation
Certificate of Achievement
Appendix A: Worksheets
Appendix B: Activities and Materials

Orders and information:
GerstenWeitz Publishers
8356 E. San Rafael Dr.
Scottsdale, AZ 85258
Phone: (480) 951-9707   Fax: (480) 993-2169
E-mail: info@speechbooks.com
www.helpmetalkright.com

How to Teach a Child to Say the "S" Sound in 15 Easy Lessons

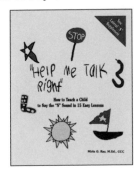

This "Help Me Talk Right" book focuses on the "s" sound. It presents an easy to follow, proven step-by-step method of frontal and lateral lisp correction. All the tools and techniques you need for "s" sound correction are included.

Free of technical jargon and easy to use, this book is for speech pathologists, speech assistants, and parents who wish to teach a child how to say the "s" sound and use it in conversation. Everything you need to know about teaching a child to say and use the "s" sound is clearly shown in a step-by-step format. Each lesson builds upon the successes of previous lessons so that the child is challenged to use the "s" more often until he is able to use it in conversation. The book comes complete with worksheets, suggestions for games and fun exercises, and a certificate of achievement.

Contents

Orders and information:
GerstenWeitz Publishers
8356 E. San Rafael Dr.
Scottsdale, AZ 85258
Phone: (480) 951-9707   Fax: (480) 993-2169
E-mail: info@speechbooks.com
www.helpmetalkright.com

Notes

About the Author

Mirla G. Raz, a certified and licensed Speech-Language Pathologist, lives and works in Scottsdale, Arizona, USA. In her long career, she has worked with a variety of speech and language disorders in her family centered clinic and in public school settings. Her popular *Help Me Talk Right* series of books have been used by 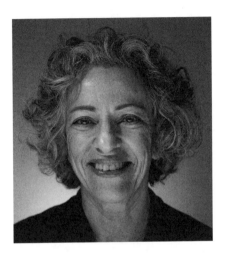 parents and professionals throughout world. Her keen interest in communication disorders and communication technology is shared with others in her blog that can be found on her website, www.helpmetalkright.com. Ms. Raz has two grown daughters and lives in Scottsdale, Arizona with her husband and two dogs.

Notes